Practical
Exercise Therapy

To our students
who, in learning from us,
teach us so much

Practical Exercise Therapy

Margaret Hollis
MBE MCSP DipTP
Formerly Principal, Bradford School
of Physiotherapy

With contributions by

Barbara Sanford
DipPE(Lond. Univ.)
Lecturer in Physical Education
Bradford School of Physiotherapy

Patricia J. Waddington
MCSP DipTP
Principal, School of Physiotherapy
Manchester Royal Infirmary

SECOND EDITION

Blackwell Scientific Publications

OXFORD LONDON EDINBURGH
BOSTON PALO ALTO MELBOURNE

© 1976, 1981 by
Blackwell Scientific Publications
Editorial offices:
Osney Mead, Oxford OX2 0EL
8 John Street, London WC1N 2ES
9 Forrest Road, Edinburgh EH1 2QH
52 Beacon Street, Boston
    Massachusetts 02108, USA
706 Cowper Street, Palo Alto
    California 94301, USA
99 Barry Street, Carlton
    Victoria 3053, Australia

First published 1976
Reprinted 1977
Second edition 1981
Reprinted 1983, 1984

Set in 11 on 12 point Baskerville

Printed and bound in Great Britain at
the Alden Press, Oxford

DISTRIBUTORS

USA
Blackwell Mosby Book Distributors
    11830 Westline Industrial Drive
    St Louis, Missouri 63141

Canada
    Blackwell Mosby Book Distributors
    120 Melford Drive, Scarborough
    Ontario M1B 2X4

Australia
    Blackwell Scientific Book
    Distributors
    31 Advantage Road,
    Highett, Victoria 3190

British Library
Cataloguing in Publication Data
Hollis, Margaret
    Practical exercise therapy.–2nd ed.
    1. Physical therapy
    I. Title   II. Sanford, Barbara   III. Waddington,
    Patricia J.
    615.8′2   RM725

IBSN 0-632-00806-7

Contents

Preface

This book was long on my mind, but was an impossible proposition if I could not find colleagues to deal with two aspects of exercise therapy so ably described by my two collaborators. The spectrum of therapeutic exercise is too wide to be encompassed in detail by one mind without a tendency to bias in a particular field.

Opportunity to write the book arose after Miss Waddington and I had just discovered we could amicably write technical material together. With Mrs Sanford I have worked closely for many years. Without their cooperation and participation this book would not have been a feasible proposition and I am most grateful for their agreement to write their sections and to share their great expertise and wide experience so that a balanced book might be produced.

A deliberate decision was made by all of us to exclude lists of exercises and muscle work. Had we included them, in the former case we would have left nothing to the imagination and inventiveness of the reader and in the latter case we would have had to lay down the precise mode of performance of each exercise. Muscle work is dependent on how work is performed and can be analysed by observation, palpation or electrical recording. In the second edition I have, however, shown how muscle work should be analysed, but readers will have to go to other source books for analyses of specific exercises or remember previous learning and widen their present knowledge by analytical observation, experiment and recording.

As hydrotherapy is described in recently published books we have still excluded it and at the moment I do not feel that traction is within the compass of this book—there are many others that deal with it very adequately.

It has, however, been heartwarming to learn that the first edition has enjoyed such worldwide sales and use, and in response to requests we have modified some chapters and have amplified where we thought it necessary. An entirely new section has been included on the use of large apparatus. Circuit training has been expanded and provides sample tables of exercises for fixed time and fixed apparatus circuits. Sections on mixed ability groups and on exercises and safety for wheelchair patients have been added. The book has proved to be so basic that little fundamental alteration has been needed and in the neurophysiology not at all.

Many people have helped us. Three of our students were models. Jill Nicholas, MCSP, DipTP, not only draft typed Miss Waddington's section of the book but acted as model, adviser and reader for many of our chapters and deserves our thanks.

I owe a deep debt of gratitude to Ralph Stohlner, MSCP, DipTP, who helped me with the mechanics chapter and whose meticulous attention to my grammar was both limitless and pitiless. Barbara Turner, MSCP, DipTP, also read many chapters and made helpful suggestions, as did many other colleagues too numerous to mention who were asked for opinions, comments and criticism. Dr M. W. Arthurton, MD, FRCP, DCH, Consultant paediatrician in Bradford, kindly read and critically advised me about the section on exercises for babies and infants. Without the generous help and encouragement of all these people the book would never have reached final form.

Mrs Muriel Cawthra has deciphered and typed the alterations for this edition and I am grateful for her patient work.

Finally the staff of Blackwell Scientific Publications Limited have encouraged us at all times and I am grateful for their interpretation of my diagrams, so creating more realistic illustrations and for their organization of the new material, the revisions and the original text into a coherent new edition.

Margaret Hollis   *Bradford 1981*

Acknowledgements

I am grateful to the following companies who lent me photographs.

Carters (J & A) Ltd for Figures 128, 129, 130 and 133 of their walking aids.

Electro Medical Supplies for Figures 124 and 125 of their Rehabilitation Unit.

Portabell Keep Fit Systems Ltd for Figure 143B.

Rank Stanley Cox for Figure 71 of the Guthrie Smith Suspension Frame and Figure 137 of their Variweight Boot.

Our photographers were Mrs V. Cruse of Pudsey, Mr P. Harrison AIMBI of Bradford and Mr R. E. S. Murray AIIP of Manchester to whom we owe our thanks for their patience and their expertise.

Miss Waddington wishes to thank the late Miss M. Knott BS, FCSP (Hon.) of the Kaiser Foundation Rehabilitation Center, Vallejo, California and Dr Karel and Mrs Berta Bobath FCSP of the Western Central Palsy Centre, London for the theories and techniques she learned while studying their courses.

CHAPTER 1

Introduction

M. HOLLIS

The application of therapeutic exercise to a patient is a process which demands an initial examination of the patient's needs and a constant reassessment of the situation in the light of progress or retrogression. It also demands a knowledge of the condition from which the patient suffers, the potential recovery rate and complications which may arise. In addition the therapist must constantly bear in mind the anatomy of the part being treated and of the whole body; the physiological reactions of the body to all exercise and the particular exercise she is applying at the moment, and the underlying mechanical principles associated with the exercise and/or techniques applied.

Therapeutic exercise is also influenced by a psychological reaction in which the patient may or may not wish to get better. If he wishes to improve he may be overeager to please and do too much or perform badly and in haste. If he does not wish to improve it may be because he is afraid. He may be in pain and fear more pain, he may be afraid his illness or accident may recur, or he may have a fundamental fear of the whole field of medicine and hospitals in particular.

This barrier must be overcome and a rapport established between patient and therapist so that the therapist may initiate the proceedings which will eventually lead to the patient achieving his maximum independent potential.

To this end a few simple but important rules should be followed by the therapist. First, each patient should be known by name and greeted and welcomed at each treatment session. Secondly, fear of more pain can be overcome by working and teaching on parts which are not painful. Each action should be taught on the soundest or least painful part, then on the afflicted part gradually working towards the part he most dreads having treated. In this way he will not only be reassured but there will probably be less pain due to facilitation of inhibition. As he relaxes he will relax his protective painful spasm and so have less discomfort.

Thirdly, his activities must always be harnessed to a goal which is within his potential of achievement. This has two uses; it is a goal for which he can strive and a matter for congratulation when achieved. The objective can be reset each day or each week or with no regularity at all, but it is most important that the early goal is remarked upon when achieved as then the patient will gain confidence in his therapist as well as in himself.

It is said that initially patients have a 'love–hate' relationship with their therapists. This may be so as the therapist may have to insist on the patient performing an uncomfortable manoeuvre and he will not be grateful for it until some time has elapsed. Examples of this situation arise when a patient with an

1

ineffective cough must be persuaded to cough more effectively to void his chest secretions in spite of the pain of his abdominal incision; and when patients have to contract the quadriceps muscle group following knee surgery. In both these cases patients freely admit later on that they hated the therapist at the time, but are grateful now that they were persuaded to do their therapeutic exercise.

Therapists who work in this climate become accustomed to this attitude from their patients and learn to use all their manual and psychological skills for the improvement of the patient.

With the patient who has a long-term problem, short-distance goal setting is even more important, and knowledge of the medical history of the patient, his social background and his home and work environment will be necessary to determine the sequence of the goals to be achieved. Personal independence should usually be aimed for initially. This may be toiletry, personal care and dressing, feeding or ability to get about. Some go hand in hand. It is no use being able to undress and dress in the toilet if there is no possibility of physically getting there.

It is essential that the therapist gradually withdraws what she does for the patient so that eventually he does every task for himself. If this goal cannot be achieved then it is important to recognize that substitution must occur, e.g. if independent walking is unsafe and not improving the patient must come to terms with the appropriate walking aid. Recognizing the moment when no further progress is being made is as important as the first assessment of a patient. Failure to recognize this fact leads to false hopes on the part of the patient and his family and a waste of the resources of the therapist, the tools of her work and the patient's time and effort.

TYPES OF MUSCLE WORK

There are two main ways in which a muscle may work. It may contract and produce no movement, called isometric contraction, or it may produce movement during contraction, called isotonic contraction.

Isotonic contraction

When a muscle works isotonically it contracts and the part of the body to which it is attached will move. There are two types of isotonic contraction.

Isotonic shortening

When a muscle performs a contraction and its two attachments are approximating to one another, the contraction is known as an isotonic shortening, e.g. when the arm is raised from the side and the abductors of the shoulder contract, the contraction is one of isotonic shortening.

Isotonic lengthening

When the attachments of a muscle move slowly away from one another and the muscle allows this movement to occur in a controlled manner, the muscle action is one of isotonic lengthening, e.g. when the body is in the upright position and the arm is lowered from abduction to adduction, the abductors of the shoulder will control the movement and these abductors will be acting in isotonic lengthening.

Isotonic shortening can take place under any circumstances, i.e. whenever movement takes place in which the attachments of a muscle approximate the muscle work will be isotonic shortening. Isotonic lengthening, however, may only be brought about if an outside force is applied to the component which is to be moved and the body part is slowly moved so that the attachments of the muscle are moved away from one another. Gravity may be the outside force which pulls body components towards the earth as in lowering the arm from the abducted position to the side, or in sitting on the edge of a table lowering the outstretched leg to a right angle at the knee. However, under many other circumstances, in order to work a muscle in isotonic lengthening it is necessary for the therapist to be the outside force. The command given is '*resist slightly whilst I move your leg*', or arm as the case may be, to a new position. The patient offers slight resistance, the therapist applies pressure which is greater than the resistance offered by the patient and is on the surface which is on the same aspect as the muscles which are required to be worked in isotonic lengthening. For example, if a patient is in Side Lying and the quadriceps are to be worked the leg will be arranged straight at the knee, one hand will be placed as a stabilizing hand on the thigh and to palpate the quadriceps. The other hand will be placed on the anterior aspect of the leg and the command will be given '*resist slightly while I bend your leg*'. The patient resists, the therapist bends the leg and the quadriceps will be worked in isotonic lengthening.

Many other examples of isotonic shortening and isotonic lengthening can be found and therapists should attempt to work out the single movements of each of the joints of the body with and without resistance so that they are able to identify isotonic shortening and isotonic lengthening. When therapists can identify these two types of muscle work they should then try to apply the range of muscle work as described below.

Isometric contraction

When a muscle works isometrically it shortens its muscular length and slightly lengthens its noncontractile components and in doing so no movement occurs at any of the joints over which that muscle passes. It is easiest and in fact usual for an induced isometric contraction to be performed when a muscle is resting at the innermost part of its range, i.e. with the muscle attachments approximated, but with practice the skill can be developed so that it is possible isometrically to contract a muscle or muscle group at any part of the range. Isometric contraction can be taught to a muscle by the application of a manual resistance which is exactly equal to the contraction which the muscle produces. The command which the therapist will give will be '*don't let me push or pull that body component about*', e.g. '*don't let me push you forwards*' with pressure on the back of the shoulders will initially cause contractions of the extensor muscles. '*Don't let me pull you back*' will cause contraction of the flexor muscles. '*Don't let me push your foot up*' will cause contraction of the plantarflexors of the foot. '*Don't let me push your foot down*' will cause contraction of the dorsiflexors of the foot. When isometric contractions are done to one group of muscles only, they are usually taught in order that the patient might practice these contractions alone without the therapist. Indeed isometric contractions are the only contractions which are possible when the patient is wearing a support such as a plaster or a fixation splint. This is the type of muscle work which is used when the joint is so inflamed that movement would be both painful and inadvisable. The strength and tone of the muscles working over that joint may be maintained by teaching the patient isometric contractions. When a patient is initially incapable of performing an isometric contraction on a damaged part, the technique may be taught on the opposite limb or may be taught on any part of the patient, and if this is completely impossible the contraction *per se* may be taught with the use of a faradic type current applied in such a manner that it merely teaches the patient what to do and is immediately followed by patient participation. In other words the current is used for reeducation of contraction.

Range   The word range may be used in two senses. First, it may refer to the amount of movement which occurs in a joint. Secondly, it may refer to the amount of shortening or lengthening of a muscle as it acts to produce or control movement.

Range of movement at a joint   This is the total quantity of movement when a joint is moved to its full extent. The names of the movements are those anatomical names which are normally applied (see Chapter 4) and the method of recording range is well laid down in the book *Joint Motion* published by the American Orthopaedic Association.

One may measure and record the amount of range of movement in a certain direction, e.g. the range of abduction of the shoulder joint is 90°. The range of adduction of the shoulder joint is 90°. This is normal range. If, however, the range is limited the available range can be recorded when a zero starting point is necessary and the recording could be from 10° of abduction to 80° of abduction, i.e. the first 10° and last 10° of movement are absent and the available range is 70°.

Muscle   When a muscle contracts and performs a movement it is said to have acted through a certain range. When a muscle is fully stretched and contracts to the limit of its normal capacity it is described as having contracted and produced a movement in *full range*. For purposes of description full range is broken down into three components which overlap (Figure 1).

Outer range of contraction is from full stretch of the muscle to mid point of the full range. Inner range of contraction is from the above-mentioned mid point to full contraction. Middle range of contraction is any distance between the middle of the outer range and the middle of the inner range. Middle range of contraction is that in which many muscles work most of the time when they are producing movement.

Extreme inner range is more difficult to perform because it requires a contraction of a greater number of motor units of which a muscle is composed and usually also the muscle is pulling with an adverse angle of pull which diverts some of the effort to distracting the two joint surfaces.

Extreme outer range is also difficult because usually the angle of pull is adverse and some of the effort is diverted to compressing the two joint surfaces and, in addition, the muscle may have to overcome inertia and be working against a long or heavy weight arm. It is possible when some movements occur that in moving from full outer to full inner range, with the body in certain positions, gravity may resist the movement when outer range is performed and assist the movement when inner range is performed. When this occurs then the same muscles will not be working throughout the range of movement. The last part of the range of movement (gravity assisted) will be controlled by the antagonists working in their outer range but working in isotonic lengthen-

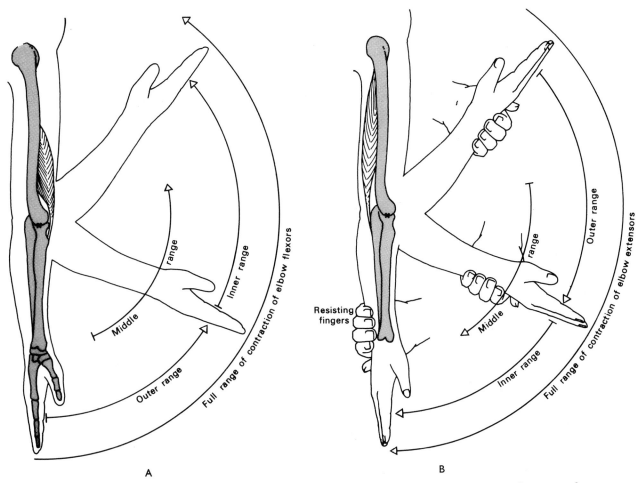

Figure 1   A, The range of movement produced by contraction of brachialis. Gravity resisting; B, The range of movement produced by contraction of triceps. Manually resisted.

ing. It is thus possible to describe muscle work by mode of action, i.e. type of muscle activity (isotonic shortening or lengthening or isometric) and, in the former case, to describe the range of the muscle work (Figure 2).

Group action of muscles

Muscles do not work in isolation. They must, for smooth coordinated movement to occur, operate in one of the following roles.

Prime movers or Agonists   In this case they are those muscles which initiate and perform movement.

Antagonists   These can produce the opposite movement to that produced by the Agonists.

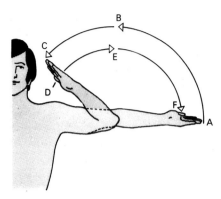

Figure 2 In the movement from A–B the elbow flexors are working in isotonic shortening in outer range (resisted by gravity); from B–C the elbow extensors are working in isotonic lengthening in outer range (pulled by gravity). In the movement from D–E the elbow extensors are working in isotonic shortening in outer range (resisted by gravity); from E–F the elbow flexors are working in isotonic lengthening in outer range (pulled by gravity).

When the Agonists work the Antagonists must relax reciprocally, i.e. exactly an equal amount. The tension of the Agonist contraction is equalled by the relaxation of the opposing muscles in order to allow smooth movement to occur.

Synergists   These are muscles which contract in order to bring about a joint position to make the action of the Agonists stronger. They most frequently may be observed in action when the Agonists are bi- or multi-axial muscles, e.g. the wrist extensors. Synergists also contract to prevent extra or additional movements that the Agonists might otherwise perform. They operate from unconscious levels.

Fixators   These muscles also operate from unconscious level to fix the attachments of the agonists, antagonists and synergists. This does not mean that they fix a component of the body and keep it there throughout the whole of one particular muscle action; rather their role is dynamic as is that of the synergists. Fixator muscle work probably constitutes about 75% of normal daily muscle action. Their role is not isometric except for very short periods, it becomes isotonic in alternating patterns so that movement is smooth. In the example quoted above the fixator muscle work would be those around the elbow to fix the forearm and hand, the shoulder to fix the arm and shoulder girdle and of the remainder of the body to fix such parts as are not totally supported. The fixator muscle work of an action such as threading a needle will be very different from that in throwing a heavy ball, both in quantity and quality. In the former case the starting position may be sitting and therefore the fixator work will be confined to those muscles which maintain the sitting position and the shoulder girdle and arm muscles involved in a fine pincer grasp and approximation of thread to needle.

In the case of throwing a heavy ball, the fixator work will change rapidly as the body prepares for and carries out the throw followed by a braking action to prevent loss of position or balance.

TYPES OF MOVEMENT

Movement takes place at joints and is brought about by either the patient's muscular efforts or by the application of an external force.

Movements may be classified as passive or active.

Passive

Passive movements are those brought about by an external force which in the absence of muscle power in the part may be mechanical or via the therapist.

a Mechanical—the pull of gravity causing 'flopping'.

b The therapist performing movements. The therapist may produce accessory or anatomical movement at joints.

Accessory movements occur when resistance to active movement is encountered and fall into two types. The first type is seen when the metacarpophalangeal joints, which do not normally do so, rotate when grasping an object such as a hard ball. The rotatory movement is not possible unless resistance is encountered.

The second type of accessory movement can only be produced passively. They are produced when the muscles acting on the joint are relaxed and are those which cannot be performed actively in the absence of resistance. An example is distraction of the glenohumeral joint when the fingers are hooked under a heavy piece of furniture and the body is pulled upwards.

Anatomical movements are those which the patient could perform if his muscles worked to produce that movement. These are dealt with in detail in Chapter 6 but can be subdivided into relaxed, forced and stretching.

Active

These are performed by the patient either freely, assisted or resisted.

a Freely—in which case mechanical factors will play a part offering either resistance or assistance.

b Assisted—when the therapist adopts the grips as for passive movements and assists the patient to perform the movement. The disadvantage of assisted active movements is that it is impossible for either party to detect how much work is being performed by each of them.

c Resisted—when mechanical or manual resistance is applied. The mechanical resistance may be in the form of weights, springs, auto loading or the mode of performance of the activity.

All these types of movement are described in the ensuing chapters but it must be remembered that the human being is subject to most of the laws of mechanics and to physiological factors which make it able to react to stimuli in accordance with the state of development of the neuromuscular system and with the integrity of both the mechanical and neuromuscular systems of the body. A broken bone, a torn ligament, a ruptured muscle, damage to the nervous system will each have their detrimental effect on the normal activity of the body.

In some of these cases rest may be an essential prerequisite to recovery with the consequent deterioration in muscle power, in others the muscles will react in an abnormal manner due to the abnormal impulses impinging on the central nervous system.

It is not the intention of this book to outline all the rapidly advancing frontiers of knowledge of the present day in respect of the neuromuscular system nor of the well understood mechanics of normal motion, but a fundamental study of anatomy, physiology and mechanics must proceed at the same time as this text is being used.

CHAPTER 2
Applied Mechanics

M. HOLLIS

Some understanding of the action of forces on bodies and of the reactions of the human body to the application of forces is essential if the therapist is to comprehend the factors which will assist or resist human motion. This chapter does not set out to deal with all the mechanical principles in detail, but should be studied along with a standard textbook on mechanics. Mechanics may be defined as the science of forces acting on bodies and the resultant effects.

Matter is anything that occupies space. There are three states of matter, the solid of which the human body is an example; liquid, which we enter when using a pool, as in pool therapy; and gas, with which we are surrounded the whole time as air. The majority of movements of the human body occur from a solid object such as a chair through air to perhaps another solid object or merely through air from one area to another.

Consideration must now be given to the mechanical laws related to motion.

Newton's first law of motion

This states: 'If a body is at rest it will remain at rest and if it is in motion it will remain in motion at a constant velocity until acted on by a force.'

If an object is moving in a straight line at a constant speed it is in equilibrium, but in the absence of a propelling force it will gradually come to a halt due to the action of forces in the form of air resistance and friction. This law is the law of inertia.

Inertia is the property of a body by which it opposes any change in its state of rest or of motion. A body possesses an inherent tendency to remain at rest or in motion due to its inertia. The inertia of a body is directly proportional to its mass and it may be said that the mass of a body is the measure of its inertia. A stationary body will remain at rest indefinitely unless acted upon by a force. A moving body will continue to move with the same velocity until acted upon by another force. If adequate force is applied to a stationary body it will cause movement and the degree of acceleration will be proportional to the force applied and in the direction in which the force is applied. When muscles are extremely weak, they may be able to contract but unable to overcome the inertia of the part on which they act. In this case the therapist will need to initiate the movement and the weak muscle made to maintain it. Once the movement has been initiated the patient may not only maintain it by the application of further force in the direction of the movement already occurring but may be able to stop the movement by contracting the opposite muscle or by ceasing to contract the muscle group originally working.

Force is that which alters the state of rest or motion of a body. A force has four characteristics. They are:

a   Magnitude.
b   Action line.
c   Direction.
d   Point of application.

To describe fully a force all four are necessary as to alter any one of them is to alter the effect of the force.

A single force applied to a body which is free to move may cause movement in the direction of the force, e.g. one muscle group will cause movement in one direction if the contraction is great enough (Figure 3,A). Two

forces applied in the same direction and at a common point are equivalent to a single force acting in that direction and at that point (Figure 3,B). The magnitude of the force applied is equal to the sum of the magnitude of the individual forces. Determining the single force that would produce the same result as a number of separate forces is known as the *composition of forces* and the single force is referred to as the *resultant force*.

Two equal forces acting along the same action line but in different directions will cause movement of an object in the direction of the greater force (Figure 3,C). Two equal forces acting on an object and in opposite directions will result in a state of equilibrium (Figure 3,D).

Parallelogram of forces states that when two forces act on a body at the same point from two different angles the body will move in a direction which will be the diagonal of a parallelogram drawn from the point of application (Figure 4). Many examples of this occur in the muscular arrangements of the body, e.g. Deltoid by its arrangement. The result will be seen when two people hit a ball simultaneously at the same point as in shooting at and defending a netball ring. The shooter strikes the ball at one angle, the defender may strike at the same point and the deflection of the flight of the ball will be in a direction between the two angles of striking.

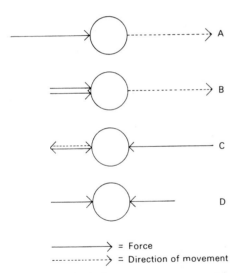

———————⟩ = Force
------------⟩ = Direction of movement

Figure 3   A, A single force causes movement in the direction of the applied force; B, Two forces applied at the same point and along the same action line cause movement equivalent to the magnitude of the sum of both forces; C, Two forces of unequal magnitude acting in opposite directions will cause movement in the direction of the greater force; D, Two forces of equal magnitude applied in opposite directions will cause a state of equilibrium. In each case the length of the line represents the magnitude of the force.

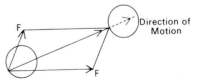

Figure 4   The parallelogram of forces—movement of an object occurs along the diagonal of a parallelogram when two forces act at the same point but in different directions.

All the other laws relating to force may be illustrated by using a ball. If a ball is rolled along level ground it will roll in the direction in which the force is applied for a distance which will be related to the frictional resistance of the surface on which it is moving and the air resistance, and will continue to travel until the energy which was originally imparted to the ball is lost. If a heavier ball is rolled with the same mechanical energy applied it will travel a shorter distance or if more mechanical energy is applied to the ball it will travel for a greater distance. If a large ball is taken and two people simultaneously apply finger tip pressure to the ball, the ball will roll a distance which is the equivalent of the sum of the energy imparted by the two people who pushed at the same time. If two people push on opposite sides of a ball and their push is equal then the ball will remain stationary between their hands.

Velocity is speed in a particular direction and will change if the force producing the movement is altered. If the force is increased the body will move with increased velocity, i.e. it will accelerate. If the force is reduced the velocity will decrease, i.e. it will decelerate.

Speed is the rate at which an object moves and can be measured in kilometres per hour. Speed is uniform if an object travels the same distance during every second that it is moving, but speed can be variable according to the forces which are acting on the moving object. Muscles can contract faster or more slowly to vary speed of motion of the part on which they act.

Natural speed—each individual has a natural speed and rhythm at which they find it easier to perform motion. Natural rhythm should be used to make work easier for a patient and variations in speed and rhythm should be used to make work more difficult. Reduced speed requires great muscular effort and more control. Increased speed requires stronger effort and momentum is thereby gained.

Gravity is the pull which the earth exerts upon all objects within its gravitational field.

Mass is the total quantity of matter a body contains. It is a fundamental property of matter and does not vary.

Weight is a secondary and variable property, it is in fact a measure of the gravitational pull of the earth on a body.

Gravity is the force by which all bodies are attracted to the earth. The earth has a gravitational field in which this force acts. The force decreases with the height above the earth's surface, in fact diminishes as the inverse square of the distance. The weight of an object depends on two factors, the mass or quantity of matter it contains and the gravitational attraction the earth has for it.

$$W = M \times g$$

Where W is the weight, M is the mass and g is the pull of gravity. If you go far enough above the surface of the earth you get outside the earth's gravitational field and become weightless.

When the weight of a part is fully supported the pull of gravity is counterbalanced, but the pull of gravity may be used to resist muscle work, e.g. when any part of the mass of the body is moved away from the earth. When movement of any part of the mass of the body towards the earth occurs then gravity will assist the movement.

Centre of gravity is the point in a mass at which all forces operate. The centre of gravity of the erect human body lies at about the level of the second sacral vertebra, and light pressure applied with one finger tip to

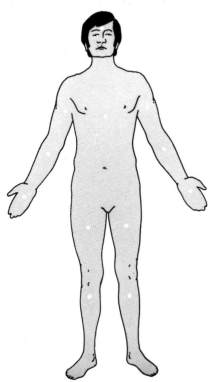

Figure 5 The centre of gravity of each body component lies at approximately the junction of the proximal and middle one-third.

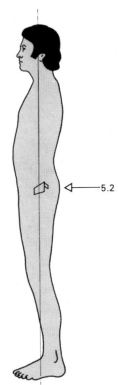

Figure 6 The centre of gravity of the standing human body is at the level of the second sacral vertebra. The line of gravity falls from the vertex, through the centre of gravity, in front of the ankles and within the base.

this point will cause the body to move forward. Pressure applied to the side of the buttock at the same level will cause the body to move sideways. This is a key point at which pressure must be exerted to help a weak patient to stand upright. It is a 'locking' point (Figure 6) at which assisting pressure must be exerted to maintain a patient upright. The centre of gravity of each of the parts of the human body lies at about the junction of the proximal and middle one-third of each body component (Figure 5).

Line of gravity is a vertical line which falls through the centre of gravity and within the base. When the human body is in the standing position the line of gravity passes from the vertex through the second sacral vertebra to just in front of the ankle joint and between the feet (Figure 6).

The relationship of the various body structures to this line is subject to considerable variation in accordance with posture and anatomical structure, but for balance to be maintained it is essential that the line from the centre of gravity should fall within the base (Figure 6).

Base is the area which supports a body or object. In the case of a chair it is the area of

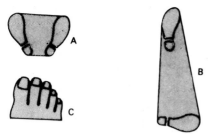

Figure 7   A, The base in Stride Standing; B, The base in Lunge; C, The base in Standing on one tiptoe.

and within the chair feet. In the case of the human body it is the area supporting the body, e.g. in Standing it is the area of the feet and the space between them (Figure 7).

The larger the base the more likely is the line of gravity to fall within the base. Thus a person lying down has a very large base and a person standing on the tiptoe of one foot has the smallest possible base while still remaining on the floor. In both these cases equilibrium will be maintained only if the line of gravity falls within the base and the centre of gravity is therefore also over the base.

Equilibrium is present when the forces acting upon a body are balanced and the body remains at rest. There are three types of equilibrium.

Stable equilibrium   If the forces acting on a body tend always to restore it to its original position after it has been displaced, the body is said to be in stable equilibrium. The most stable position of equilibrium is when the centre of gravity is as low as possible and the line of gravity falls near the centre of an extensive base. This is so when the body is in the Lying position.

Unstable equilibrium occurs if, when a body is given an initial displacement, the forces acting upon it tend to increase the initial displacement. This occurs when the centre of gravity is very high, the base is very small and the relationship between the two is difficult to maintain. Unlike inanimate objects which would fall over if displaced, the human body is able to maintain a position of unstable equilibrium by the activity of muscles. The more unstable the position the greater the muscular activity required. This can be clearly demonstrated by comparing the amount of reflex muscle activity as seen in the movement of tendons around the ankle when a person stands on two feet and then on one foot. An extreme example of this would be to stand with upstretched arms on tiptoe. A very small displacement of the arms would cause the equilibrium to become unstable. To maintain balance, a foot would be moved to widen the base and prevent the body from toppling or leaning.

Neutral equilibrium   If in spite of displacement of a body the height and position of the centre of gravity remains the same, the body is said to be in neutral equilibrium. This occurs in a rolling ball on a plane surface and may occur in the human body when it is being rolled as in performing passive or active medial and lateral rotation of either the upper or lower limb with the patient in the Lying position.

Newton's second law of motion

This states: 'When a force acts on a body it produces acceleration which is proportional to the magnitude of the force and inversely proportional to the mass of the body.' This is the law of acceleration.

Acceleration is the rate at which the change in velocity occurs. If an opposing or braking force is applied the body may lose its velocity and come to a halt.

The sudden application of opposite or braking force will bring the part to an immediate halt. Deceleration in a movement may indicate the onset of fatigue and also occurs when a patient inhibits a movement due to pain or the contraction of the antagonists, or alternatively if the agonists (prime movers) are insufficiently strong to complete the movement.

Momentum is the total quantity of motion possessed by a moving body and is expressed as:

$$\text{Mass} \times \text{Velocity} = \text{Momentum}$$

e.g. thus a wheelchair containing a heavy patient requires a greater braking force to bring it to a halt than does a pushchair containing a child provided they are moving at the same speed.

Once movement is initiated, use is made of momentum to decrease the effort by increasing the speed of movement. The effort is increased when the speed of movement is decreased as then momentum is of less assistance. In this way work may be graded and the effect of changing the rhythm of movement can be most easily estimated when the number of repetitions of an exercise per minute is counted and graded. When there is an increase in the number of repetitions of correct performance of an exercise, there is thus progressive effort which is greater.

Newton's third law of motion

This states: 'To every action there is an equal and opposite reaction.'

If a body *A* exerts a force on a body *B*, body *B* exerts an equal and opposite force on body *A*. A book presses down on a table and the table exerts an equal pressure on the book.

When standing, force is exerted through the sole of the foot; the supporting surface pushes upwards against the sole of the foot. The ground presents a reaction force equal in magnitude and with the same action line to the downthrust of the foot (Figure 8).

In the diagram R_1 represents 'heel strike', R represents the 'stance phase' and R_2 represents 'toe off' in walking. R_1 and R_2 are

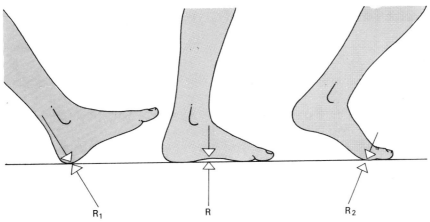

Figure 8 R_1 represents 'heel strike'. R represents 'stance phase' when the pressure downwards equals the pressure upwards. R_2 represents 'toe-off'. In R_1 and R_2 there is a horizontal component to the thrust.

both greater than R due to the momentum of the forward moving leg in R_1 and to the thrust imparted by the calf muscles in R_2. In R the position is briefly stable as the floor pushes vertically upwards. In R_1 and R_2 there is a horizontal component to the force which must be opposed by an equal and opposite force so that the foot is stable. This counter force is provided by friction.

Friction is the force which tries to stop one object from sliding over another. The force of friction has the quality of adjusting its magnitude to that of the force tending to produce motion within certain limits. Friction may be *static friction* which tends to prevent movements or *kinetic friction* which is the friction between one body moving on another surface. Kinetic friction is obviously less than static friction, the coefficient of static friction is higher than that of kinetic friction which reduces if the two surfaces moving on one another are more highly polished. There are two types of kinetic friction.

Sliding friction is the resistance experienced when two parts slide on one another.

Rolling friction is the friction exhibited when a wheel moves forwards and makes a slight impression on the surface on which it is moving.

Friction is greater on irregular surfaces and some materials are more adhesive and offer greater frictional resistance than others. Without friction it would be impossible for us to walk about. The feet or shoes must be able to grip the surface before we are able to progress in any direction. If friction is minimal the body will tend to counteract this, e.g. when walking on ice short steps are taken to allow a downward pressure on the slippery surface, because a normal pace and 'heel strike' will cause the 'striking' heel to skid.

The same will happen to the rear foot on toe 'push-off'. This is another example of Newton's Third Law: 'To every action there is an equal and opposite reaction'. But if friction is great the body will tend to reduce the friction by reducing the surface contact or alternatively will try to work on an inclined plane. Examples of the use of more friction are between the ferrules of crutches and sticks and the floor: between the brakes and wheels on a wheelchair and between the patient and the bedclothes either when attempting to move or to turn. When giving lumbar or cervical traction the surface on which the patient lies should have a high coefficient of friction. It is usually provided by strapping the underblanket and sheet to the plinth top. An example of rolling friction is between the wheels of a wheelchair and the floor. Examples of reducing friction are in using a formica table top or well powdered piece of hardboard used as a polished board to slide a limb about, or in suspension as the round rings of the hooks provide a minimal frictional surface and the body part is removed from the drag of the bedding. In using absorbent powder such as Biosorb when moving one body part on another, e.g. in massage, friction is also reduced.

Energy is defined as the capacity to do work and therefore the energy possessed by a body is the measure of the work it is capable of doing. There are two types of mechanical energy—kinetic energy and potential energy.

Kinetic energy is the energy of motion. A body has kinetic energy because of its velocity or speed of motion.

Potential energy is the energy of position.

These are called respectively K.E. and P.E. illustrated in Figure 9 which shows a pendulum. The weight on the end of the cord is lifted

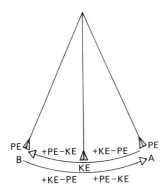

Figure 9 A pendulum demonstrating kinetic and potential energy.

i.e. they may be pulled out to a greater length, as in a spring, than their resting length, in which case they will have gained potential energy, stored in the stretched spring.

Recoil occurs when the potential energy is used to restore the extended elastic body such as a spring to its original shape. As the spring recoils the potential energy is converted to kinetic energy.

to position A and whilst it is held there it has potential energy. When it is released and begins to fall it gains kinetic energy and loses potential energy. As it passes through the lowest point of its arc of motion the energy is entirely kinetic. As it rises towards point B it loses kinetic and gains potential energy until at point B the energy is again entirely potential (Figure 9). The pendulum will continue to oscillate in this way until the energy originally imparted to it as a result of the work done in lifting the weight has been used up in frictional losses.

Elasticity A body which is able to regain its original form or shape after it has been distorted by the application of a force is said to be elastic. The force applied to an elastic body is known as *stress* and *strain* is the quantity of change in size or shape. The relationship of stress to strain is stated in **Hooke's Law** which says: 'The strain is proportional to the stress producing it' (so long as the elastic limit is not exceeded, when permanent deformity of the elastic body will occur). Materials which are elastic also have the property of extensibility,

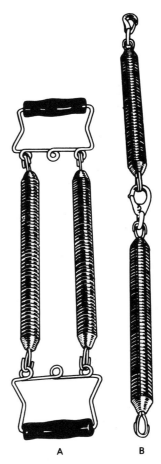

Figure 10 A, Springs in parallel; B, Springs in series.

Some modern materials such as silicone putty have the property of plasticity in that they can be deformed by pressure and will offer considerable resistance to the deforming force. However, such materials return slowly to their original shape or may spread out if left on a flat surface or move downwards if left on an inclined plane. They do not return to their original shape after being deformed.

The 'weight' of a spring   The mean coil of the wire and the wire diameter can be varied so that springs can be made to offer different quantities of resistance expressed in pounds or kilos which is usually noted on the tab at the end of the spring. The full resistance which is offered by each spring is reached when the cord inside the spring is on full stretch.

Springs in parallel   If two springs are arranged side by side attached to the same point, i.e. in parallel, the weight of the resistance will be the sum of the two (Figure 10, A).

Springs in series   When two springs are joined end to end, i.e. in series, the resistance offered is the same as if only one spring is used, e.g. if two 10 kg springs are attached end to end the resistance offered will be 10 kg, but the range through which movement must occur to stretch two springs fully would be twice as great (Figure 10, B). If the same range as would be required to stretch one spring fully is considered then the force applied to the two in series would be half the weight resistance of one, i.e. 5 kg. Connecting springs in series, therefore, is indicated if either the range over which the springs must stretch is great or a spring of sufficiently low weight resistance is not available.

CHAPTER 3
Simple Machines

M. HOLLIS

LEVERS

A lever is a simple machine consisting commonly of a rigid bar which pivots about an axis called the fulcrum. It may enable a large weight to be moved by the application of a relatively small force. When the force is less than the weight moved the lever is said to have a mechanical advantage of more than one.

Mechanical advantage is the number of times the lever increases the force applied, i.e. it is the ratio of the load to the effort.

The weight moved is referred to as the *load* (symbol W) and the force producing the movement is called the *effort* (symbol E).

$$\text{Mechanical advantage} = \frac{Load}{Effort} \text{ or } \frac{W}{E}$$

Consider Figure 11 as follows:

A.F. is referred to as the *weight arm*.
B.F. is referred to as the *effort arm*.

The moment of a force is its turning effect and is expressed as the product of the force and the distance from its point of application to the fulcrum. In the example in Figure 11 the anticlockwise moment of W about F is equal to $W \times A.F. = 10 \times 4$. An effort of 10 applied to B would exactly balance this and fractionally over 10 would raise the load. The mechanical advantage in this case

$$\frac{W}{E} \text{ or } \frac{10}{10} = 1.$$

But if the fulcrum is moved so that the length of the effort arm $B.F.$ exceeds that of the weight arm $A.F.$ then a mechanical advantage of more than one is gained because in the balance lever shown in Figure 12

$$W \times A.F. = E \times B.F.$$
$$(10 \times 3 = 30) = (6 \times 5 = 30)$$

Therefore the mechanical advantage is $W/E = 10/6 = 1.67$. The effort required to move the same weight is much less.

In applying a knowledge of levers to the human body it must be remembered that the bones represent the rigid bar, the joints are the fulcra and the muscles provide the effort. Since the muscle attachments are fixed in their distance from the fulcrum (joints) it is only

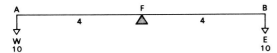

Figure 11   A balance lever showing the moment of force and a mechanical advantage of one.

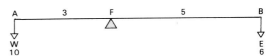

Figure 12   A balance lever showing a mechanical advantage of 1·67.

17

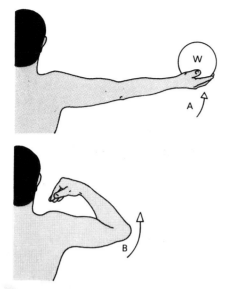

Figure 13   A, A long weight arm; B, A short weight arm.

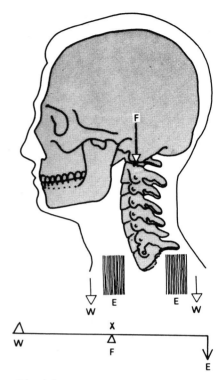

Figure 14   A human example of a lever of the first order (balance).

possible to alter the length of the weight arm or the weight of the load (Figure 13).

There are three orders of lever.

The first order of lever is one of balance as described above with the fulcrum in between the weight and the effort. In the human body a balance lever is found when the head nods on the atlanto-occipital joint. The fulcrum is this joint. The weight is alternately the back and front of the skull and the effort is alternately the flexors and extensors of the head. (Figure 14).

The second order of lever is one of *power* in which the fulcrum is at one end of the rigid bar, the effort is at the other end of the bar and the weight is in the middle. As the weight is nearer the fulcrum than the effort, the effort arm must always be longer than the weight arm. Consequently levers of the second order always have a mechanical advantage greater than one with the result that the applied effort

is less than the weight to be moved. An example of this type of lever is flexion of the elbow using brachioradialis when the forearm is in mid pro and supination and provided no load is held in the hand (Figure 15,A). Another example is when the foot is pushing off the ground in the 'heel-off' phase of walking (Figure 15,B). The weight falls in front of the ankle, the metatarsophalangeal joints are the fulcra and the power is provided by the muscles inserted into the tendocalcaneus. This type of lever results in a powerful movement which is often slow.

The third order of lever is one of *speed* when the fulcrum is again at one end of the rigid bar, with the weight at the other end and the

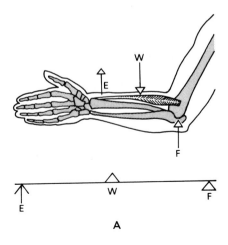

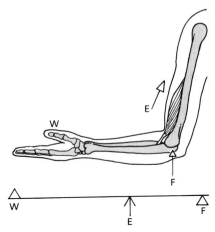

Figure 16 A human example of the third order of lever (speed). Flexion of the forearm by brachialis.

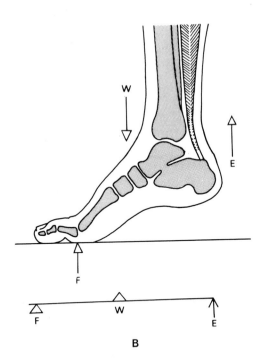

Figure 15 Human examples of levers of the second order (power). A, The action of brachioradialis in flexing the forearm; B, The foot pushing in the 'toe-off' phase of walking.

effort between. Since the length of the weight arm always exceeds that of the effort arm the mechanical advantage is less than one and a force or effort greater than the weight of the load must be applied, more so if the effort is very near the fulcrum and the weight arm is considerable. A small movement of the nearer point of the lever brought about by the effort results in a large range movement of the more distant weight, but the effort required to perform this movement will be great. The extra force required is compensated for by the gain in speed. This is the commonest order of leverage in the human body (Figure 16).

PULLEYS

A pulley is a simple machine and either gives a mechanical advantage or changes direction of pull. It consists of a grooved wheel which pivots about an axial pin, encased in a block (Figure 17). The pin and pulley are usually metal and the block is often made of artificial fabric. To one end of the block is usually fastened a clip device while the other end has

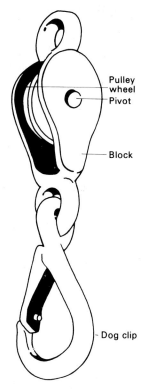

Figure 17 A pulley.

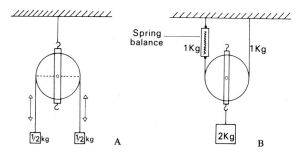

Figure 18 A, A pulley demonstrating that it serves to change the direction of the force; B, A pulley suspended to show how the load is distributed at the suspended points.

a ring attached. Either end may be the means of attaching the pulley to a fixed point, but the spring clip is more commonly used as it usually has a pivoting pin which allows rotational adjustment and prevents the rope from chafing.

A single fixed pulley has a mechanical advantage of one as the load on the pulley wheel requires an equivalent force to allow it to be balanced. Such a pulley serves to change the direction of the force which must be applied in order to move the load (Figure 18,A). Use is made of this simple device in the reciprocal pulley circuits described in Chapter 10 and also in the rope and pulley circuits which allow combined oblique and rotary movements.

A multiple pulley circuit offers a greater mechanical advantage than a single pulley. This is demonstrated if a pulley with a weight attached is inverted and hung from a hook in the ceiling by a cord, and a spring balance is inserted into the cord circuit to measure the force (Figure 18,B). Each side of the cord takes half the weight and therefore the mechanical advantage of the circuit will be two.

If a second pulley is inserted into the circuit so that a downward pull can be applied to the cord then the mechanical advantage is unchanged. The ceiling still takes half the weight at each suspension point, but the rope can now be moved. As it moves the loaded pulley will move upwards, but the rope will travel twice the distance that the load will move. In Figure 19 the rope C remains stationary but shortens, rope B moves up and over pulley P_2. Rope A lengthens by the distance pulley P_1 travels up the rope A and the distance rope B travels over pulley P_2. The load of 1 kg on pulley P_2 balances the load of 2 kg on pulley P_1.

The advantage of the use of two pulleys

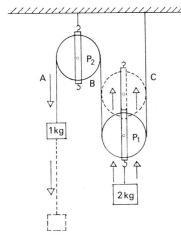

Figure 19 Demonstrates the mechanical advantage offered by inserting more than one pulley in a circuit.

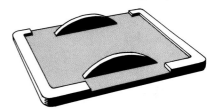

Figure 20 A square 'Wobble' (Balance) Board offering a means of varying the stability of the surface on which the patient stands.

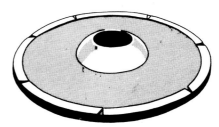

Figure 21 A round 'Wobble' (Balance) Board offering greater instability than that shown in Figure 20.

is seen in the double pulley rope in Figure 77, p. 68. Here not only is there a mechanical advantage of two, but the therapist pushes the cleat *down* the rope thus performing a gravity-assisted movement.

A multiple pulley circuit with a mechanical advantage of one is used to change the direction of pull as seen in Figure 126, p. 101.

COORDINATION OR 'WOBBLE' (BALANCE) BOARDS

These are boards made of 2 cm thick wood covered with a 0·75 cm layer of rubber with a non-slip surface.

The boards are made in three shapes:

a Square, 56 cm (Figure 20).
b Oblong, 56 cm × 102 cm.
c Round, diameter 56 cm (Figure 21).

The undersurface of the board has screwed to it an attachment as follows:

a and **b** Two sections of a cylinder of a height of 5 cm with a length of 20 cm fixed, in the case of the longer board, parallel with the long side so that when rocked this board gathers more momentum than the square board. In each case the segments of the cylinder are placed about 10 cm from the edge of the board and equidistant from the other two edges.

c One section of a cylinder of a diameter of 20 cm and a depth of 5 cm is placed centrally, the central part being flat and the peripheral part being bevelled.

In using these boards the progression is made by first using the square board, then the oblong board and finally the round board.

The aim is to stand in the centre of the board and keep it still by using all the postural muscles and balance reactions. At first it may be necessary to stand in front of wall bars or between parallel bars and hold on, then let go with one hand and then the other. These boards were originally designed by Mr M. A. R. Freeman MD, FRCS, for treatment of functional instability of the foot, but their use is now much more extensive than this as their mechanical and physiological value has been recognized. Their use is recommended in the chapter on balance (Chapter 27). They can also be used in cases of instability of the knee and hip.

Full-length coordination board

This is a board on which a patient may lie and to accommodate most people, needs to be made of wood 20 mm thick, with a width of approximately 610 mm and a length of approximately 2000 mm.

Rockers are placed across the two ends as in the small oblong board, but the higher the centre of the rocker the greater the tilt which can be operated. As these boards are tilted by the therapist to bring about balance and 'righting' reactions in neurologically disabled patients, care must be taken either to tilt them by their ends or to have finger grips bevelled out of the sides so that the therapist does not trap her fingers. (See Chapter 26.)

CHAPTER 4

Fundamental and Derived Positions

M. HOLLIS

There are five fundamental positions which are usually described along with their derivatives as the starting positions from which exercises start or in which they may be given.

Muscle work is deliberately not described as it is dependent upon the way in which the body components relate to one another. It must be recognized that maintenance of position is dependent on the integration of interplay of isotonic muscle action and of some isometric muscle work, but once a position has been assumed the body will reduce its muscle work to the minimum necessary to maintain that position. The abbreviations for each word are also provided.

Lying (Ly.) or Supine (Sup.) The body is supine with the arms by the sides and legs straight. This is the position in which the body is most supported with a large base and low centre of gravity.

Sitting (Sitt.) The body is erect, arms by the sides, the thighs are fully supported and together. Right angles are maintained at the hips, knees and ankles. The centre of gravity is low but near to the rear edge of the base which is the area between both the legs of the seat and the feet.

Kneeling (Kn.) The body is upright from the knees which are held at a right angle. The arms are by the sides. The base consists only of the legs and the centre of gravity is high and the line of gravity falls close to the edge of the base, making the position unstable and difficult to maintain.

Standing (St.) The body is erect with arms by the sides. The feet are slightly apart at the toes. The base is small and the centre of gravity is high. Providing the lower limbs are strong this position is easier to maintain than kneeling.

Hanging (Hg.) The body hangs from a beam or overhead support. The arms are wide apart (more than shoulder width) and should be braced so that there is no undue traction on the shoulders. This position should only be used for very strong people as the base consists of the hands grasping the beam and supporting the full body weight.

Positions derived from Lying

Side Lying (S.Ly.) This position is rarely used as turning onto the side with the under arm by the side and legs straight is very difficult both to perform and to maintain. The base is small and rounded and the position is one through which the body passes in turning movements or is modified by bending the under arm and leg forwards while the upper arm and leg either rest in the straight position or are flexed slightly. This position is then

23

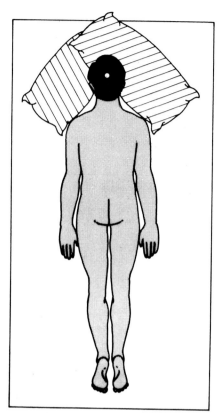

Figure 22   Prone Lying.

called the Right Lateral position (lying on the right side) (R.Lat.) or Left Lateral position (lying on the left side) (L.Lat.).

Prone Lying (Pr.Ly.) or Prone (Pr.)   The body is face down with arms by the side and legs straight. In order to rest comfortably two pillows should be crossed (Figure 22) to support the forehead or the head allowed to turn to the side of the patient's choice.

Across Prone Lying (Acr.Pr.Ly.)   Lying across a support with the anterior superior iliac spines just off the front edge of the support (Figure 23). The head and hands may rest on the

floor, or be in line with the legs according to the exercise to be performed. The feet should be held by a partner or support from a wall bar.

Quarter Turn (¼ Tn.)   The body is turned through 45° from either Lying, Side Lying or Prone Lying and supported by pillows down the raised side of the trunk. The direction of the ¼ turn is indicated by stating the starting position and direction, e.g. ¼ Tn.L. from Ly.

Half Lying (½ Ly.)   The body is bent at the hips and the trunk is raised from lying to any angle up to 90°. This is the standard position in which most sick people are propped up in bed (Figure 58, p. 51). More comfortably the legs may be slightly raised or lowered from the horizontal and the knees bent. This modified position is achieved by using ergonomically designed beds or by placing a pillow under the knees.

Side Half Lying (S.½ Ly.)   The trunk and head are turned to one side so that the patient rests on one buttock and leg and that side of the trunk (Figure 61, p. 52).

Positions derived from Sitting

Forward Lean Sitting (Fwd.Ln.Sitt.)   The trunk is inclined forwards and the head is supported on pillows on a table at the front.

Half Sitting (½ Sitt.)   Sitting on the side of a seat so that only one buttock is supported. The leg on the side of the unsupported buttock is usually bent at the knee as this position is used when the hip is stiff in extension or for lower limb above-knee amputees to allow exercise of the stump (Figure 24).

Long Sitting (Long Sitt.)   The legs are stretched out in front, knees straight. The trunk is

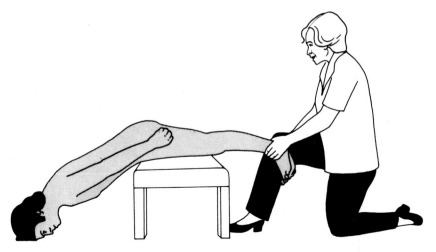

Figure 23   Across Prone Lying.

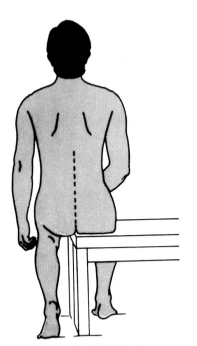

Figure 24   Half Sitting.

upright and the position is an uncomfortable one to maintain.

Positions derived from Kneeling

Kneel Sitting (*Kn.Sitt.*)   From kneeling to sitting back on the heels. A stable position and much used for retraining balance and by children at play.

Side Sitting (*Side Sitt.*)   From kneel sitting the buttocks are moved sideways so that one or both buttocks rest on the floor beside the feet (Figure 25).

Half Kneeling ($\frac{1}{2}$ *Kn.*)   From kneeling, one leg is taken forward to be bent at right angles at the hip, knee and ankle. A stage in rising from kneeling to standing or transferring from floor to stool.

Prone Kneeling (*Pr.Kn.*)   Kneeling supported by all four limbs. The arms should be straight and the hands in line below the shoulders.

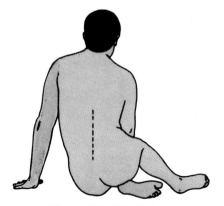

Figure 25   Side Sitting.

Right angles should be maintained at the hip and knee and the ankles may be plantar-flexed or dorsiflexed (Figure 26).

Positions derived from Standing

High Standing (High St.)   Standing on a platform or stool of any height. Normally used when one leg is to be moved and allows the patient to be more accessible to the therapist. The position is usually stabilized by allowing the patient to grasp a support.

Step Standing (Step St.)   Standing with one foot on a higher level than the other. Used for teaching weight transference before walking upstairs (Figure 27).

Half Standing ($\frac{1}{2}$ St.)   Standing on one leg, i.e. one hip is hitched up or one leg is bent at the hip and knee.

Close Standing (Cl.St.)   The feet are together and parallel. Harder to maintain than standing not only because the base is slightly smaller but because the axes of the ankle joints are no longer at an angle to each other, but together form a single long axis which results in increased interplay of muscles in front of and behind the joints.

Toe Standing (T.St.)   The body is raised onto the toes. The smallest possible base is now in use.

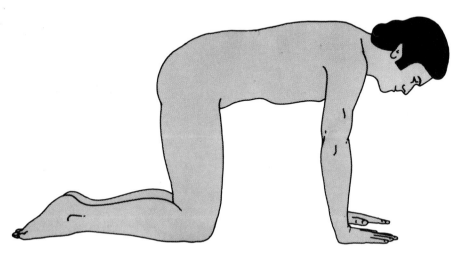

Figure 26   Prone Kneeling.

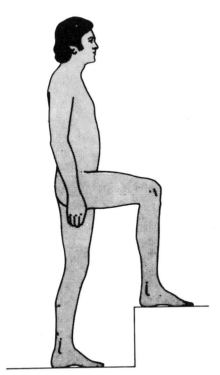

Figure 27   Step Standing.

Positions derived from Hanging

Arch Hanging (*Arch Hang.*)   The starting position for forward and backward swinging of the trunk or for bar somersaults.

Half Hanging ($\frac{1}{2}$ *Hang.*)   Hanging by one arm. The position achieved during lateral travel on the beam.

Positions derived by moving the Arms (*A*)

Any of these may be incorporated into the fundamental positions or into those derived from them.

Half ($\frac{1}{2}$)   One arm.

Stretch (*Str.*)   The arms are held straight above the head in the position of elevation (flexed and laterally rotated) at the shoulder, i.e. palms facing inwards.

Yard (*Yd.*)   The arms are held straight out from the side of the body, palms facing downwards (Figure 100).

Reach (*Rch.*)   The arms are held straight in front of the body palms facing inwards (Figure 101).

Head rest (*H. Rst.*)   The hands rest on the head, more usually on the occiput, and the position is usually used to gain upper trunk extension (Figure 94,B).

Bend (*Bd.*)   The elbow is bent and the hands lie adjacent to the shoulders. A starting position usually used for thrusts upwards, forwards, downwards and backwards.

Wing (*Wg.*)   The hands rest on the hips. Little used except in rotatory movements of the trunk when the arms are fixed and the quantity of trunk movement is therefore limited.

Heave (*Hve.*)   Usually used with a grasp. The arms lie abducted at the shoulder, the elbows bent upwards at a right angle so that

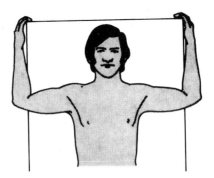

Figure 28   Heave Grasp.

a grasp may be taken of the edges of the bed or plinth. Used to fix the upper half of the body (Figure 28). Alternatively may be used as Heave Hanging

Grasp (*Gr.*)   The hands grasp a convenient support. May be used with Stretch, Yard, Reach or Heave (Figure 86, Figures 100 and 101).

Low Grasp (*Low Gr.*)   The hands grasp when they are by the sides.

Forehead Support (*F.head Supp.*)   The forehead rests on the hands placed either palm down or with loosely grasping thumb and forefinger (Figure 29). Used in Forward Lean positions.

Arm Lean (*A.Ln.*)   The forearms and the hands palms down are placed on a support in front of the body, the head may rest on them or they may rest on and be covered by a pillow on which the head rests. Used in Forward Lean positions (Figure 59).

Forward Propping (*Fwd.Prop.*)   The hands rest flat on the seat and in front of the trunk.

Backward Propping (*Bwd.Prop.*)   The hands rest flat on the seat fingers pointing backwards and behind the trunk (Figure 126).

Reverse Propping (*Rev. Prop.*)   The hands rest as above but the fingers point forwards. All three propping positions are used for thrusting actions in which the arm is braced in extension and the trunk may be balanced and/or moved on the arm/s.

Positions derived by moving the Legs (*Lg*)

Stride (*Std.*)   The feet are a sideways pace apart and the base is therefore wide from side to side giving good lateral stability.

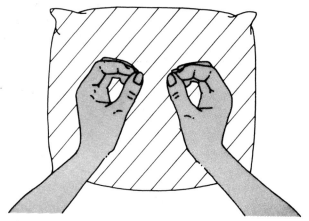

Figure 29   The loosely grasping thumb and forefinger resting on a pillow ready to receive the forehead for Forehead Support.

Walk (*Wk.*)   The feet are a forward pace apart and the base wide from front to back giving good anteroposterior stability.

Oblique Stride (*Obl.Std.*)   The feet are a pace apart part way between walk and stride. This position allows oblique transfer of weight.

Lunge (*Lge.*)   The feet are well apart and at right angles to each other. If the rear leg is bent then the weight is in a back lunge position. If the front leg is bent the weight is in a forward lunge position. This position allows transfer of body weight from one leg to the other, with maximum stability for working in this position.

Step   One foot is supported on a stool of any height. The weight may be on either the rear or the stepping foot.

Crook (*Ck.*)   The knees and hips may be bent slightly by using one pillow under the knees or, in the extremely flexed position, the soles of the feet will be flat on the support (Figure 30).

Cross Leg (X Leg)   The legs are crossed at the ankles. The knees are flexed and the hips flexed, abducted and laterally rotated. This position is taken up on the floor or on a high mat.

Cross Ankle (X Ankle)   The legs may be crossed at the ankles when the body is in the Lying, Sitting, Kneeling or Standing positions.

Positions derived by moving the Trunk (*Tr.*)

Stoop (Stp.)   The body is bent forwards at the hips with erect back and head.

Relaxed or Slack Stoop (Lax Stp.)   The head and trunk are flexed.

Arch   The head and trunk are extended (Figure 115).

Turn (Tn.)   The trunk is rotated through any degree less than 90° either by moving the shoulder girdle or the pelvis or both depending on the fundamental position (Figure 89).

To describe a position

First consider which parts of the body are not in the normal relationships as in the fundamental position. Then name their position in the following order—Head, Arm, Trunk, Leg and fundamental position, e.g. Head Support Arm Lean Forward Stride Sitting; ½ Low Grasp ½ High Standing.

DESCRIPTIONS OF MOVEMENTS

Flexion (Flex)   An angular movement. A forward movement in which joints are bent. Usually the approximation of two ventral surfaces. Takes place about a transverse axis and in the median or sagittal plane.

Extension (Ext.)   An angular movement, the

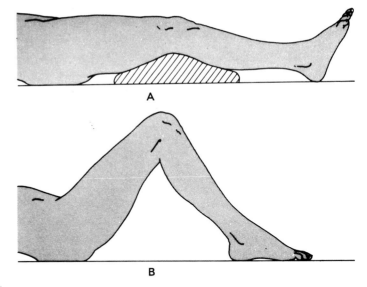

Figure 30   A, Crook Lying using a pillow for flexing the knees; B, Crook Lying with the knees so flexed that the feet are fully supported.

opposite of the above. A backward movement in which joints are straightened. The opposite of flexion with the same axis and plane.

Abduction (Abd.)   An angular movement. Movement away from the mid-line of the body, occurs round an anteroposterior, i.e. sagittal axis and in the coronal or frontal plane. The exceptions are the shoulder joint and the carpometacarpal joint of the thumb.

Adduction (Add.)   An angular movement, the opposite of the above. Movements towards the mid-line of the body.

Circumduction ○   A combination of the above four angular movements so that each position is adopted in turn and in sequence. The moving bone/s circumscribe a conical space.

Rotation (Rot.)   A turning movement, about a vertical axis and in a horizontal plane, of limbs, head or trunk in which case the direction in which the anterior surface is turning is first indicated.

Medial Rotation (*M.Rot.*) Occurs round a vertical axis. The anterior aspect of the limb turns towards the mid-line.

Lateral Rotation (*L.Rot.*) The opposite of the above, though the axis is the same.

Side Flexion (*S.Flex.*) An angular movement. Movements of the head or trunk away from mid-line in a lateral direction.

Inversion (*Inv.*) Applies to the foot and is a movement of adduction and inward rotation of the forefoot of which the sole faces inwards.

Eversion (*Ev.*) Applies to the foot and is the opposite of the above.

Supination (*Sup.*) Applies to the forearm. The palm of the hand is turned forwards so that the thumb is lying laterally.

Pronation (*Pron.*) The opposite of the above. The movement is limited to the radio-ulnar joints and best observed when the elbow is flexed. (Neither of the above should be confused with Medial and Lateral Rotation of the Arm.)

Symbols, apparatus and counts

⊙ *Circling* may be a movement of a part involving all four angular movements and rotation and the term may also be used to describe an action by a group of people.

○ *Circumduction* consists of a composite of the four angular movements with no intention to rotate.

⤴ R.L. ⤴ *Rolling* in direction of arrow.
→ Movement in that direction, viz. ↑ up, ↓ down, → R. to the right, L. ← to the left, ⫽ obliquely.

(Form) (Stool) etc. placed in the exercise name after the fundamental position.
4 × repeated four times.
1–4 to a count of 4, may be followed by an indication of tempo 1–4 (slowly).
Reb. with a rebound.
·/. repeat.

To describe an activity

First name the starting position (see above) then the part to be moved in the activity or movement.
    e.g. T. turn or Jump on spot.
Next name the direction.
    e.g. T. turn R. and L.
The apparatus to be used is named in brackets after the starting position.
    e.g. Std. Sitt. (Stool).
The repetition number and count is named after the action and is followed by the tempo description if needed.
    e.g. Std. Sitt. (Stool); T. turn alt. R. and
        L. (4 ×),
    or Std. Sitt. (Stool); T. turn alt. R. and
        L. (1–4) slowly (5–8) quickly,
    or Std. St. T. turn alt. R. and L. with reb.
        (1–4) and T. drop fwd. (5) T. Str. up.
        (6–8).

To analyse muscle work of an exercise

Watch the whole performance and observe which are the moving body parts. Then decide the joints which are moving and the direction of movement at each joint. Remember that direction may be conditioned by movement of the body part either proximal or distal to the joint. e.g. There is rotation of the cervical spine in the action of walking but the head does not move; the rotation is of the vertebral column *below* the head. Next decide on a starting point in the analysis. Most actions are both repetitive and cyclical and thus a starting point is needed so that a decision can be made about the exact part of muscle range being used at any one time. For convenience repetitive actions are often divided into phases described by what is being done at the time, e.g. in walking each leg repeats stance, toe or push-off, swing-through and heel-strike phases; one leg doing stance while the other performs the movement sequence. In throwing a ball the phases are conditioned by the starting position and the vigour of the throw as well as the size and weight of the ball and may be swing back, swing forward and release for the throwing arm, while the other arm may swing in opposite directions to assist balance and the rest of the body may be doing weight on back leg, weight transfer forwards, weight on forward leg with the upper trunk rotating with the throwing arm against a lower trunk rotated with the weight transfer.

The next decision that has to be made is: Which are the working muscles over each joint in a sequence? The same sequence should be used to name and describe the different phases of the activity. Thus the muscle groups working over the foot, ankle, knee and hip should always be described in that order if that is the order used for the first part of the analysis and description.

Each time a muscle group is named the type of muscle work it is performing and the range of muscle work should be stated, e.g. the muscle work of the swing phase of the leg in walking may be described in two ways, either

the dorsiflexors of the foot isotonic short-ening in full range; the extensors of the

knee isotonic shortening in inner range; the flexors of the hip isotonic shortening in outer range;

or

because the phrase isotonic shortening applies to all groups mentioned this phrase can be used at the end of the sentence thus—

the dorsiflexors of the foot in full range, the extensors of the knee in inner range and the flexors of the hip in outer range, all in isotonic shortening.

Recognize that at the same time another part of the body may simultaneously be doing something else and that action should be analysed next and recorded so that a synchronous picture and analysis is built up.

It must be remembered that in analysing free movement the effect of gravity will be important in determining the muscle work and will be varied mainly by the mode of performance in speed and weight. Thus trunk bending slowly forward to pick up a ball will be initiated by a momentary contraction of the flexor muscles in isotonic shortening in the middle range and brought about by the trunk extensors in isotonic lengthening in their outer range along with the hip extensors in isotonic lengthening if the hip joint is moved. In other words, in this case the *movement* is of flexion, but the muscle *action* is of the extensors.

Now if the movement is a swift and hard push into flexion the flexors will perform the action until the speed and weight of the action is reduced when the extensors will take over.

CHAPTER 5
Relaxation

M. HOLLIS

The tension of muscles can be affected by conscious effort and thought and can be relieved by the application of conscious thought and/or muscular effort on the part of the patient. The difference between tension and relaxation may be observed, for example, in the difference in posture of an athlete at the beginning of a sprint start and that at the end of the race when the line has been crossed; or in the learner driver who sits tensed and hunched over the steering wheel as opposed to the relaxation of the accustomed and experienced driver.

Relaxation can be taught to patients so that a regime can be practised alone, or active resisted techniques may be used for which the presence of the therapist is necessary. Relaxation may be general or local, i.e. the whole body may be taught to relax or only a small part, as required. Relaxation can be practised in any convenient posture, but is more usually taught in Lying, Half Lying, Side Half Lying, modified Side Lying and Right or Left Lateral positions, Prone Lying or in an armchair supported with a high back.

There are two methods, contrast method and reciprocal method, which the patient may be taught to practise alone.

Contrast method

The physiology of the contrast method is that a strong contraction of a muscle is followed by an equal relaxation of the same muscle or

$$Excitation = Inhibition$$

The technique consists of a sequence of contractions of muscles performed, usually, in a distal to proximal sequence in each limb or pair of limbs in turn followed by letting go or relaxation for an equal or longer period of time. Then the contractions for each limb part are usually added to one another so that tension in the limb is total and the relaxation should be controlled in reverse sequence.

The sequence of commands is as follows (alternative or explanatory commands are in brackets):

FOR THE ARM
'*Make a fist and let go.*'
'*Tighten your wrist and let go*' (pull your hand back or forwards).
'*Tighten your elbow and let go*' (bend or straighten).
'*Tighten your shoulder and let go*' (pull your arm into your side).

FOR THE LEG
'*Point your foot down or pull your foot up and let go*' (the patient chooses whichever is least likely to give him cramp).
'*Tighten your knee and let go*' (straighten your knees).

'*Tighten your hips and let go*' (tighten the buttocks).

When the above sequences are added together the commands will be:

FOR THE ARM
'*Tighten your fist, wrist, elbow and shoulder and let go shoulder, elbow, wrist and hand*' (stiffen the whole arm, and let go).

FOR THE LEG
'*Tighten or point your feet, knees and hips and let go your hips, knees and feet*' (stiffen the whole leg, and let go).

The commands for both pairs of limbs may be added together as follows:
'*Tighten the feet and hands, knees and elbows, hips and shoulders and let go*' in reverse order (stiffen your arms and legs and let go).

FOR THE TRUNK AND HEAD
'*Press your head against your support and let go.*'
'*Press your shoulders against your support and let go.*'
Deep breathing may be practised with relaxation of any part of the body. It is more usual to breathe in while tensing the muscles and to breathe out on letting go.

It is also possible to add the contractions for the trunk on to those for the limbs so that the patient is in whole body tension, but this should not be taught to a patient with high blood pressure, or one who tends to have respiratory incapacity. The value of this technique is that it can be used for a limited part of the body, for example, for relaxation of the hand or of the shoulder girdle or the hip adductors and lateral rotators.

Reciprocal method

The physiology of this method is that the Antagonistic groups of muscles always relax reciprocally and equally to the contraction of the Agonist groups of muscles. Tension will be relieved by contraction of the Antagonistic muscles. In this technique, the muscles which will take the patient out of the tense posture are those which are required to contract with the consequent diminution in tension in the muscles that are maintaining the tense posture.

The patient is allowed initially to remain in his tense posture, and may lie or sit if he prefers, but specially comfortable positioning should not necessarily be offered, better positions will be achieved as the relaxation proceeds. For success with this technique it is important that the patient learns to recognize his own tension at any time and learns what to do to relieve it without necessarily changing his main working position.

The sequence used is more usually proximal to distal, and each part of the body is given three commands as follows:

1 To move so that the tense '*infolded*' position of the body is opened up.
2 To stop moving.
3 To let the brain appreciate the new posture making the patient think about the new position in which his body component is now resting. Time should be allowed for this and the patient should not be hurried.

The commands are given as follows:

FOR THE SHOULDERS '*Push your shoulders towards your feet.*'
FOR THE ARMS '*Lift your arms outwards and slightly straighten your elbows.*'
FOR THE HANDS '*Make the whole palms of the hands and your fingers be fully supported.*'
FOR THE HIPS '*Separate the thighs.*'
FOR THE KNEES '*Straighten your legs slightly.*'
FOR THE FEET '*Point your feet away from you.*'
FOR THE HEAD '*Press your head into the support or backwards.*'
FOR THE UPPER TRUNK '*Press your back into the support or backwards.*'

FOR THE JAW   *'Without necessarily opening your lips push the lower jaw away from the upper jaw or towards your feet.'*

Breathing for this technique is usually achieved at greater depth by asking the patient *'to sigh'* and to appreciate what is happening to the waist. To be aware that the waist is becoming smaller, and even that the *'ribs are folding down like a bird's wing'*.

In fact in both these methods asking the patient to sigh as though at the end of a heavy day is the best method of gaining deep breathing because if a good breath out is taken the amount of air that is subsequently taken in to the lungs will be slightly increased. Note that in these two techniques the word *relax* is never used and only in the Contrast Method is the patient asked to *let go*. The positions which may be used for the Reciprocal Method are the same as those for the Contrast Method and in neither of these methods is it important that the patient should be in a particularly quiet atmosphere. It is, in fact, much better to teach the Reciprocal Method against a normal background noise and not to create a soothing hypnotic atmosphere round the patient.

Suggestion method

A third method which may be used for some patients and which is entirely suitable for those who may not perform much muscle work is the suggestion method. In this technique the therapist provides comfortable relaxing conditions for the patient:

a   A warm well-ventilated room.
b   A comfortable support.
c   Light covering.

Then, by using quiet hypnotic mellow tones, suggest that the thoughts be directed to personally enjoyable, but repetitive noises or scenes. The patient is told to think about each part of the body in turn. To think that it is *'very heavy'* and this suggestion is repeated several times until the limb gives the appearance of relaxation, e.g. until the lower limb is rolled out. The patient may be invited to try to raise the limb, while the suggestion is made that it will be impossible to do so and that it may feel as though it is floating. The patient is then instructed to direct attention to the other leg and to each arm in turn and then to the whole body. Deep, sighing type of breathing may be practised for a few breaths and the 'suggestible' patients will be found at the end of quite a short treatment session, to have gone to sleep.

Pendular swinging

This is used for relaxation of the limbs. The arm/s or leg/s may be swung back and forth until they feel numb. The sensory receptors have accommodated to the constant movement. This type of swinging may be aided by adding from a $\frac{1}{2}$ to 1 kg weight to the limb keeping it within the length of the limb, i.e. grasped in the hand, or fastened to the ankle. This type of swinging is of particular value to reduce the rigidity of Parkinsonism, but is also used for shorter periods of time to mobilize joints by patient activity. It is most suitable for the shoulder, hip, knee and lumbar spine.

Active resisted techniques for local relaxation

Hold relax

This technique is described more fully in Chapter 25 on neuromuscular facilitation. Briefly it consists of offering resistance to a muscle group which is in tension. The patient is commanded to '*hold*' the limb in position while the therapist applies resistance to the patient's contraction, which produces isometric contraction of the tense muscles. No movement should occur. When the therapist feels that the patient has reached the limit of their potential contraction, she should grasp the limb firmly, but comfortably, and at the same time tell the patient to '*relax*' or '*let go*' and allow a period of time to elapse which is at least as long as, or perhaps longer than, the time taken to build up the maximum contraction. This technique is of especial use when a patient has no movement because of pain-spasm.

Contract relax

This technique may be used when a patient has a small range of movement and then is prevented from moving further by the spasm of the muscles which are Antagonist to the movement. The therapist places her hands on the limb on the same side as the Antagonist muscles which are in spasm and asks the patient to make a small strongly resisted contraction back to the original position of rest. At the end of the movement the part is grasped firmly, but comfortably, and the patient is told to '*relax*'. Again the period of relaxation should be an adequate length of time. Then the original movement should again be attempted either passively or actively. A gain in range may be found and a further contract–relax should now allow a small range movement which should not return the limb to the original resting position, but should be less than the total range, i.e. the patient should not return each time to the original position in which the limb was resting.

CHAPTER 6
Passive Movements

M. HOLLIS

Anatomical movements which are performed by the therapist for the patient are passive movements. They may be performed at single joints or at several joints in sequence covering any or all of the joint movements and maintaining muscle length. They may also be performed to several joints simultaneously as in many natural and functional movements.

Basic rules

The following must be observed.

1 Those parts not to be moved should be adequately supported.
2 The part/s to be moved should be comfortably grasped.
3 The sequence of motion should be decided —distal to proximal or proximal to distal. Each have their place, e.g. for giving passive movements to neurological patients a proximal to distal sequence is used. The reverse, a distal to proximal sequence, is more commonly used to aid venous and lymphatic return.
4 At the extremities of the ranges, the grasp on the stretched skin side should be eased to prevent dragging.
5 The grasp should be as near the joint to be moved as possible.
6 As the movement is performed the joint may be given slight traction, but compression should be exerted at the extremities of the range.

7 The motion should be smooth and rhythmical and the repetition rate maintained at even tempo.
8 Changes in grasp should be smooth and positioning of the hands arranged so that minimal changes are necessary.

Movements of the right upper limb

Patient's position Lying (or Side Lying) The therapist stands so that she can see the patient's face and in Walk Standing with the outer leg (L) forwards. She grasps as follows.

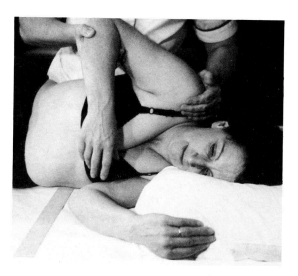

Figure 31 Grasp for elevation and depression of the shoulder girdle.

36

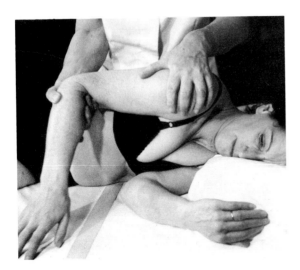

Figure 32 Grasp for protraction and retraction (lateral and medial rotation of the scapula).

Proximal to distal sequence

Shoulder girdle   There are two different grasps for:

a Elevation and depression—the left hand above the shoulder the right hand under the bent elbow (Figure 31).

b Protraction and retraction—the left hand

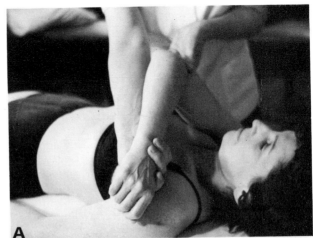

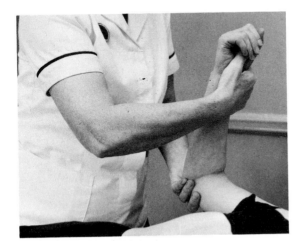

Figure 33 The grasps used for glenohumeral joint movement when the joint is not stiff showing abduction. The same grasp is used for elbow joint movement.

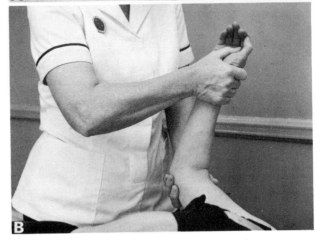

Figure 34 A, Flexion through abduction at the glenohumeral joint; B, The grasp used for medial and lateral rotation at the glenohumeral joint.

grasps over deltoid and rolls the arm and, therefore, the shoulder girdle, forwards and backwards (Figure 32).

Glenohumeral joint There are two possible grasps.

a The left hand at the elbow to grasp as in Figure 33 and to give slight traction the right hand takes a palm-to-palm thumb grasp which fixes the wrist joint in slight extension. The starting position of the arm is in neutral abduction. Movements towards the body are done first: adduction and abduction (Figure 33) then remaining in abduction (Figure 34,A) flexion through abduction and extension to the limit of the support/joint, medial and lateral rotation (Figure 34,B) follow again from neutral abduction. Full elevation follows (flexion/abduction/lateral rotation) (Figure 35).

b If the glenohumeral joint is stiff it may be necessary to fix the shoulder girdle in which case the left hand remains above the shoulder to do so. The right forearm supports the patient's arm with the therapist's hand grasping the elbow (Figure 36). The movements may be performed as above, but flexion through abduction may involve foot movement on the part of the therapist.

To complete the movements of the shoulder joint the patient should be turned into Side Lying when full extension can be performed (Figure 37).

Elbow joint The left hand grasps behind the elbow and the right hand maintains a palm-to-palm thumb grasp. Flexion is performed first, finishing with slight overpressure and extension is performed last finishing with slight traction (Figure 33).

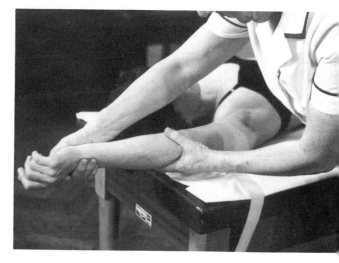

Figure 35 The grasp used to obtain full range movement into elevation of the arm (flexion/abduction/lateral rotation).

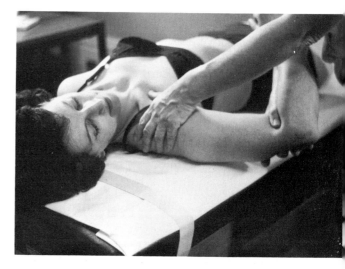

Figure 36 The grasps used to isolate the movement to the glenohumeral joint.

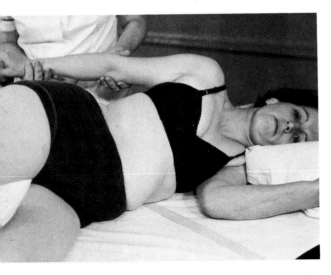

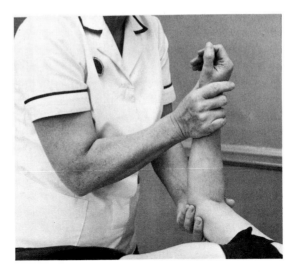

Figure 37 Side Lying grasp for full range extension of the glenohumeral joint.

Figure 38 The grasp for elbow flexion and extension.

Radio-ulnar joints The movements of pronation and supination may be performed using the same grasp as for the elbow, but to confine the movement to the radio-ulnar joint the elbow should be semiflexed (Figure 38) and kept in this position throughout the movements which follow.

Wrist joint The right hand grasps the palm and the left hand grasps proximal to the wrist (Figure 39). Flexion is performed first, being careful that the thumb on the dorsum of the hand does not drag on the skin, then extension is performed, followed by ulnar then radial deviation with the wrist in the neutral position, i.e. straight.

Thumb movements The therapist's right hand grasps the palm and the left hand grasps the thumb tip on each side (Figure 40). The movements of full flexion of the carpometacarpal, metacarpophalangeal and interpha-

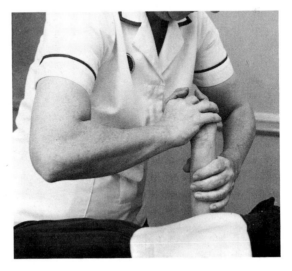

Figure 39 The grasp for wrist flexion and extension.

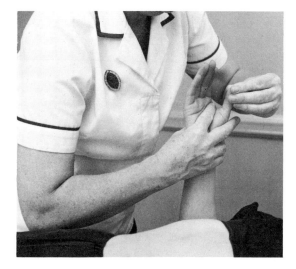

Figure 40   The grasp for movements of all the joints of the thumb.

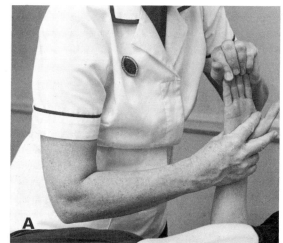

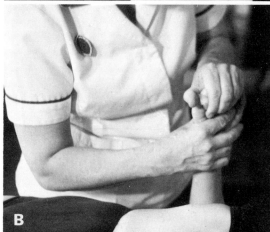

Figure 42   The grasp for A, Extension; B, Flexion of the interphalangeal joints of the fingers.

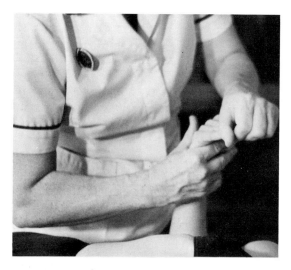

Figure 41   The grasp for movements of metacarpophalangeal joints of the fingers.

langeal joints may be performed together followed by extension, then adduction and abduction of the metacarpophalangeal and carpometacarpal joints, followed by opposition and extension of the carpometacarpal joint. Alternatively with the arm laid on the supporting pillow the movements of flexion and extension of the individual joints may be performed separately by holding the distal and proximal bone on each side and near the joint to be moved.

Metacarpophalangeal joints of the fingers The therapist grasps the palm with her right hand and the fingers with her left hand so that she

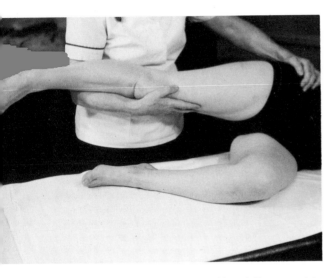

Figure 43 Side Lying grasp for full range hip extension.

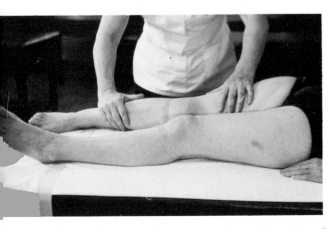

Figure 44 Grasp for medial and lateral rotation of the hip in extension.

keeps the interphalangeal joints straight (Figure 41). The movements of flexion, extension, abduction and adduction are then performed for all four joints simultaneously or with the arm laid on the supporting pillow each joint may be moved separately.

Interphalangeal joints The same grasp is maintained on the palm with the right hand and the tips of the fingers are grasped with the left hand. The fingers are bent into the palm, overpressure is given (Figure 42,A) and, as the fingers are unrolled into extension, they are regrasped at the tips so that slight traction may be given (Figure 42,B), or, again with the arms laid on the supporting pillow, each interphalangeal joint may be moved separately by holding adjacent to the joint on the sides of the bones.

Combined movements of the upper limb

a Elbow flexion with supination and extension with pronation is done to maintain the passive length of biceps brachii and the normal pattern of these two movements.
b Elbow extension with pronation and extension/abduction/medial rotation of the shoulder and its opposite elbow flexion and/or extension with supination and flexion/adduction/lateral rotation of the shoulder (elevation).
c Extension and abduction of fingers, thumb and wrist with supination and elbow extension and its opposite flexion/adduction of fingers, thumb and wrist with pronation and elbow flexion to maintain the passive length of the muscles in the anterior and posterior aspects of the forearm and working over the above joints.

Movements of the right lower limb

Patient's position Lying (or Side Lying)

Hip movements It should be recognized that full range movement of extension of the hip especially in the male cannot be achieved in **Lying**, and it may be necessary to turn the patient to Side Lying or Prone (Figure 43).

Medial and lateral rotation The therapist places one hand on the front of the lower tibial region and one on the front of the lower thigh and rolls the leg first in then out (Figure 44) or the leg may be flexed to 80° (approx.) by grasping with the left hand under the lower thigh and with the right hand under the lower leg (Figure 45). The lower leg is then moved outwards to obtain medial rotation and inwards to obtain lateral rotation. The supporting left hand maintains the flexion and allows the limb to pivot at the hip.

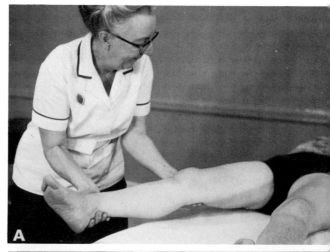

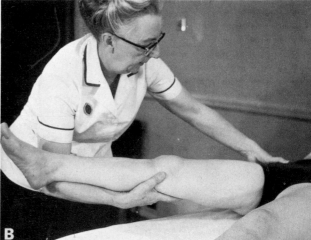

Figure 46 Alternative grasps (A and B) for adduction and abduction of the hip.

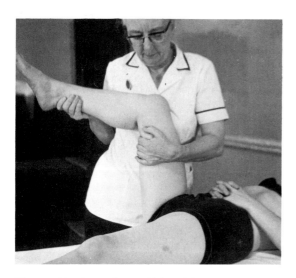

Figure 45 Grasp for medial and lateral rotation of the hip in flexion.

Adduction and abduction The therapist holds under the lower thigh with her left hand and the ankle area with her right hand with the knee slightly flexed (Figure 46,A). To permit full adduction the other leg should be abducted or the moving leg may have to be raised to slight flexion to cross in front of the opposite leg. Abduction should be carried out second and, if the opposite leg is not abducted the therapist must be careful to note when the limit of abduction is reached and the pelvis starts to tilt laterally, or the therapist holds the leg from the medial side by sliding her right hand under the knee and supports the slightly flexed leg on her forearm whilst her left hand palpates on the anterior superior iliac spine for the onset of pelvic tilting (Figure 46,B).

Flexion and extension With the patient in Lying this may be done in two ways.

a As a straight leg raise by grasping over or under the ankle with the right hand and under the knee with the left hand. The amount of

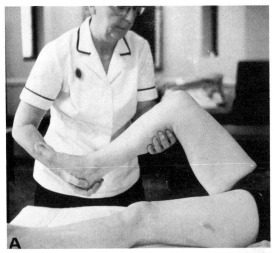

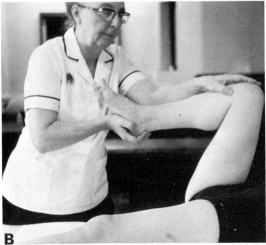

Figure 48 Hip and knee flexion and extension. A, The grasp to start and finish the movements; B, The grasp for the middle stages, i.e. full flexion and the beginning of extension.

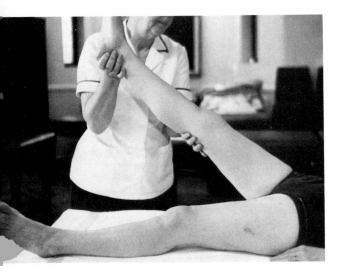

Figure 47 The grasp used for flexion of the hip by performing a straight leg raise.

hip joint flexion will be limited by the passive insufficiency of the hamstrings (Figure 47).
b With the knee flexed, when the right hand may hold under the heel and the forearm may

support the foot and the left hand holds under the lower thigh and flexion of both hip and knee joints is carried out simultaneously. To obtain full flexion with overpressure it may be necessary to move the left hand to the front of the upper tibial region as the movement passes mid-range and return it as extension starts (Figure 48).

Knee flexion and extension This can only be carried out as above if the patient is in Lying, but can be carried out alone if the patient is in Side Lying. The hip should be kept extended so that full knee extension is possible. With the patient in left Side Lying the therapist's right hand holds under the medial side of the ankle and the left hand under the medial side of the lower thigh. It may be necessary to allow slight hip flexion to occur to carry out full knee flexion because of the stretch on rectus femoris (Figure 49).

Ankle movements There are several possible grasps, in each case a pillow may be used under the calf to raise the heel off the bed.

a One hand on the dorsal and one on the plantar aspect of the mid-foot with the hands crossing the foot, fingers on the medial side. Plantarflexion should be performed first (Figure 50,A).
b The right hand takes an under heel grasp with the forearm under the foot and the left hand across the dorsum of the foot (Figure 50,B). The disadvantage of this grasp is that pressure is exerted on the metatarsal heads which may, in some diseases, cause the onset of ankle clonus. Care should be taken that the toes are not extended with unintentional vigour at the metatarsophalangeal joints.

Mid-tarsal joints Inversion and eversion can be performed by using grasp (**a**) described for ankle movements by sliding the hands more distally on the foot, or the foot may be grasped from the outside with the right hand and the left hand used across the ankle and on to the medial side of the calcaneum to stabilize the leg and proximal tarsal bones.

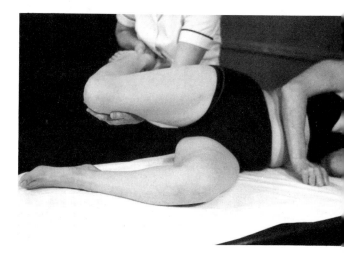

Figure 49 Side Lying. The grasp used for knee flexion and extension.

Metatarsophalangeal joints Flexion, extension, abduction and adduction can be carried out on five joints simultaneously by using the left hand to grasp the metatarsals from the inside of the foot while the right hand grasps the toes (Figure 51).

Interphalangeal joints Flexion and extension may be performed by sliding the right hand grip on the toes to the tips (Figure 52), but it is easier to deal with the lateral four toes together and the big toe separately. The grasp

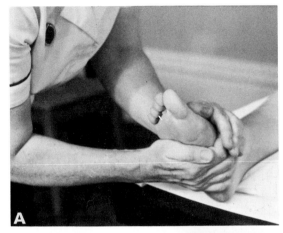

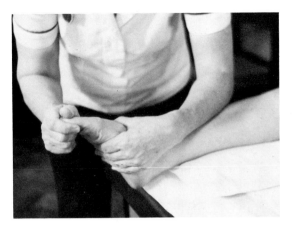

Figure 51   The grasp for all movements of the meta-tarsophangeal joints.

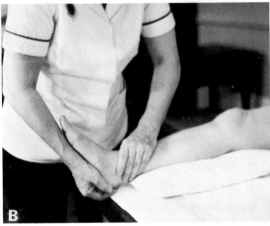

Figure 50   A, The grasp for both plantar- and dorsi-flexion of the ankle and for in- and eversion of the foot; B, An alternative grasp must be used to obtain a passive stretch on a shortened tendocalcaneous.

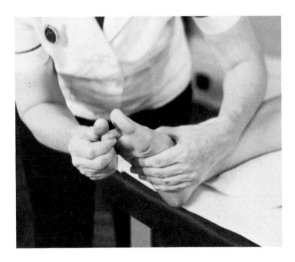

Figure 52   The grasp for flexion and extension of the interphalangeal joints of the lateral four toes.

for the big toe is with both hands reaching over the foot to grasp adjacent to the joint and on the dorsal and plantar aspects (Figure 53).

Individual interphalangeal joints of the toes may be flexed and extended by grasp on the proximal bone at the sides and the distal bone either at the sides or on the dorsal and plantar aspects.

Combined movements of the lower limb

Flexion/adduction and lateral rotation of the hip may be alternated with extension/abduction and medial rotation and flexion/abduction and medial rotation with extension/adduction and lateral rotation. In each oblique pattern of such movements the limb should be supported just about the level of the knee and under the foot and ankle.

The above movements can be combined with knee and ankle movements, those of flexion of the hip combining more usually with flexion of the knee and dorsiflexion of the ankle. Under some circumstances it is necessary to perform an extension pattern of the hip with knee flexion, especially prior to retraining a walking pattern for the 'lift off' phase of the movement.

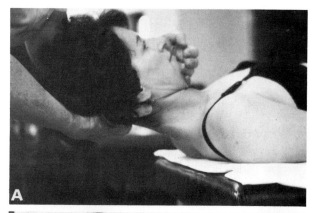

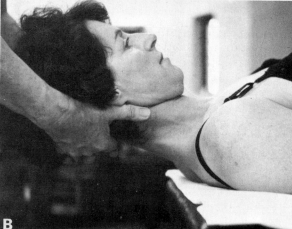

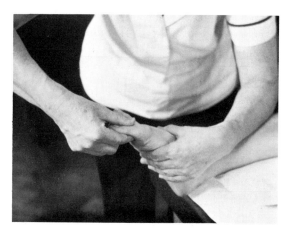

Figure 53 The grasp for movements of the metatarsophalangeal and interphalangeal joints of the big toe.

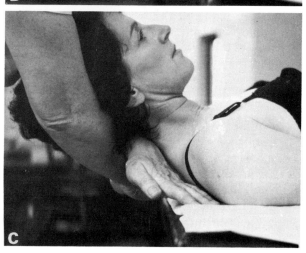

Figure 54 For movements of the head. A, The occiput and chin grasp; B, The double-handed grasp on the occiput; C, The crossed forearm support.

Foot and ankle movements often combine—dorsiflexion with inversion and plantarflexion with eversion, or dorsiflexion with eversion and plantarflexion with inversion.

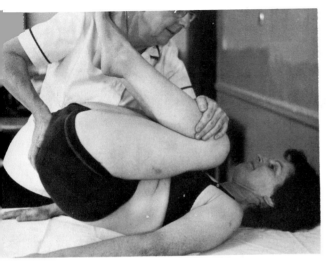

Figure 55   The grasp for lumbar flexion.

Movements of the head

Head movements may be performed with the patient in Lying with the head over the edge of the plinth and supported in the therapist's hands.

Flexion and extension   There are three alternative grasps.

a   One hand under the occiput, the other hand under the chin. The posterior hand performs the movements and gives traction. The hand on the chin keeps it 'tucked in' and controls any tendency of the head to wobble (Figure 54,A).

b   Both hands supporting the back of the head. The disadvantage of this grasp is that on full extension of the head there may be inadequate control (Figure 54,B).

c   The head is supported on the crossed pronated forearms and the finger tips rest on the front of the outer part of the patient's shoulders (Figure 54,C).

Side flexion   Grasps (**a**) and (**b**) above may be used. If the former grasp is used it may be necessary to change hands so that the head is supported at the back by the hand on the side towards which side flexion occurs.

Rotation   One hand crosses obliquely behind the head from above one ear to below the opposite ear, the other hand, at right angles to it, grasps the jaw line from in front with the fingers cupped round the chin. The head is rotated *away* from the front hand. To rotate the opposite way the hands should be changed over, moving first the front hand to support at the back and then the back hand to the jaw line.

Movements of the trunk

Passive movements of the trunk are most easily given if half the body is suspended (Figures 92, 93, 94 and 95). The unsuspended part of the trunk is further fixed by the therapist who Half Kneels behind the patient, leans across and places her arm across the front of the trunk. She braces her standing leg and uses her free arm to swing the trunk into flexion, extension or side flexion as the case may be.

If suspension is not available then the patient should be on a high mat or plinth.

To move the lower trunk

Flexion The patient is in Lying with knees fully bent and pressure is applied on the area of the tibial tuberosity with one forearm while the other hand, placed under the sacrum, lifts the lumbar spine into full flexion (Figure 55).

Side flexion The patient is in Crook Lying. The therapist hooks one arm under the knees, lifts slightly and, counter-pressing on the waist, lifts the patient into side flexion.

Rotation The patient is in Crook Lying, the therapist grasps both knees and flexing at the same time presses the knees towards first one shoulder and then to the other (Figure 56,A). Alternatively the therapist may press the bent knees to one side away from her while holding the shoulder of the opposite side still (Figure 56,B).

Extension The patient may be in Prone Lying and the therapist places one arm under the thighs and the other hand on the lumbar spine and lifts the thighs backwards (Figure 57). Alternatively the patient may be in Side Lying and the same manoeuvre may be performed by Half Kneeling behind the patient and carrying the thighs backwards supporting with one hand across the front and under the lower thigh.

To move the upper trunk

The patient may be in Stride Sitting with his arms grasped behind his neck.

Rotation The therapist stands behind and placing one hand in front of and one hand behind the shoulders she applies opposing pressures. The thigh and pelvis should be supported at the back to prevent unwanted movements occurring.

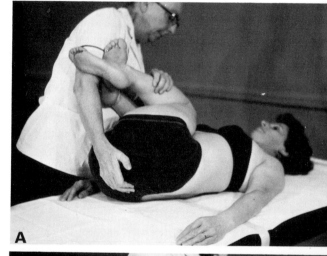

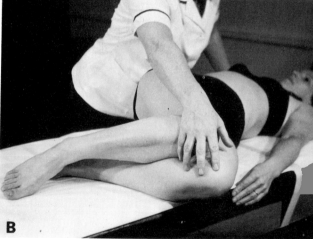

Figure 56 Alternative grasps (A and B) for trunk rotation.

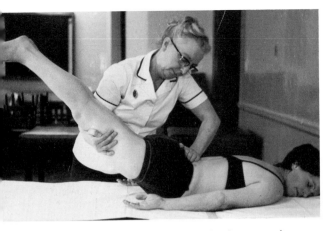

Figure 57   The grasp for lumbar extension.

Flexion   A hand is placed on the occiput and the head, neck and upper trunk are flexed.

Extension   One hand is placed on the forehead and the other in mid-thoracic region and pressure is applied to the forehead while the lower hand exerts counter pressure and also acts as the pivot.

Side flexion   The therapist stands at the back of the patient, hooks her arms from in front through his bent elbows and by levering on his grasped arms moves him from side to side.

Assisted active movements

Movements in which the patient participates but is helped by the therapist are assisted active movements. The disadvantage of such movements is that the amount of work being done by the patient is an unknown quantity and may vary considerably in the course of several repetitions or even in different parts of the range of movement.

However, in some circumstances it may be necessary to perform assisted active movements by:

a   Asking the patient to join in and perform some muscle action.
b   Initiating and completing the movement for the patient while allowing him to produce all the muscle effort he can for the easier middle range.

The grips for assisted active movement in which the patient is joining in are those for the passive movements as described earlier in this chapter.

For the second type of assisted active movement, i.e. help at the beginning and end, the same grips may be used, but for the middle range the therapist removes that half of her hand which would be the 'helping' part. Thus, the grip is maintained in the direction of the movement and sensory stimulation is only applied to the 'leading' surface.

Forced passive movements

A movement which is taken beyond the easily available range is a forced movement and there must be differentiation between over-pressure and forcing.

A forced movement to lengthen tight articular structures may be performed when the patient is anaesthetized and should only be done by a doctor who has already explored all other avenues of regaining joint range. Following this manipulative procedure the therapist may be required to maintain the required range and will have to do so in spite of the limitations of pain. The 'Slow Reversal Hold Relax' technique should be used until maximum active range has been gained and then at the limit of the present range a firm but quick extra pressure is given to regain the lost range. All the rules for giving passive movements must be obeyed in performing this technique.

Gradual stretching is another form of passive movement usually performed on either:

a Babies with congenital deformity when the basic rules for grasp and support are obeyed and the corrected position of the deformed part is achieved three times in succession followed by attempted active muscle work by reflex skin stimulation (see Chapter 18) **or**
b Those with shortened structures due to adaptive shortening. Taking the joint to the limit and applying constant overpressure will result in some lengthening under some circumstances and if associated with the application of appropriate serial plasters or splints.

CHAPTER 7

Breathing Exercises

M. HOLLIS

It may be necessary to teach breathing exercises either to improve chest expansion or to obtain better relaxation of the thorax and thus increase expiration of air. In the normal respiratory act expansion of the thorax or inspiration is active and expiration follows by the cessation of the action of the inspiratory muscles, i.e. it is passive. The thorax may be expanded in three diameters and equally relaxed in the same diameters. These are:

Vertical Brought about by the descent of the diaphragm (outer range action).

Lateral Brought about by the continued action of the diaphragm as it elevates the lower ribs pulling from the now fixed central tendon assisted by the action of the intercostal muscles. The tension of the abdominal wall prevents the unlimited descent of the diaphragm and the central tendon becomes fixed on the compressed abdominal contents.

Anteroposterior Continued action of the diaphragm causes the distal end of the sternum to move forwards, assisted by the action of the pectoral musles.

All the diameters may be expanded in quiet inspiration but additional work by the accessory muscles of inspiration can produce greater elevation of the upper ribs (lateral expansion) and greater forward movement of the sternum (anteroposterior expansion).

Relaxation of the muscles will cause the thorax to return to its resting state which is the position at the end of expiration. It is assumed that alveoli will enlarge and air will enter the parts expanded by the different muscle actions and similarly that air will be expelled on the relaxation phase.

Quiet respiration involves the movement in and out of a relatively small quantity of air 400–500 ml about 15 times a minute giving about 4 seconds for each breath. Thus when breathing exercises are taught it must be recognized that the timing of the commands and the length of time allowed for performance is important. If it is desired to increase expansion of a large part of the thorax the *rate* must be slowed down or the patient will be hyperventilated.

$$\text{volume} \times \text{rate} = \text{ventilation rate}$$
$$500 \text{ ml} \times 15 \text{ pm} = 7500 \text{ (ventilation rate)}$$
$$1000 \text{ ml} \times 7 \text{ pm} = 7000$$

Equally it must be recognized that attempts to expand a very localized area of the thorax will fail if too long a time is allowed for the effort. The patient will be attempting to direct less than 500 ml to a limited part of the thorax. In order to do this he must be given less time than is allowed for his normal breath and the moment a movement of expansion

51

starts to occur other than in the desired area he should be told to '*stop*' and '*breath out*'. In this way he can ventilate a required area and will not hyperventilate.

If the thorax has normal movements but poor muscular activity then the patient will need to be taught expansion as described later.

If the thorax rests in an expanded posture and the patient has difficulty in breathing out he is also likely to have weakness or lack of use of some inspiratory muscles, usually the diaphragm and lower intercostals, and to use the accessory inspiratory muscles for his normal breathing. In such a case expiration must be taught before correct inspiration can be achieved.

The patient should be advised to practice regularly, doing exercises for each part of the thorax in groups of six to a total of twenty-four, and attempt to practice six times a day. It is a good idea to advise practice before each meal or snack. Most people have a total of six drinks or meals a day and this frequency is more likely to be remembered than hourly.

Position of the patient

The patient should always be put into what, for him, is a relaxed position. This will vary with his capacity to relax in any position and his individual needs and difficulties.

The classical position of Half Lying (Figure 58) with the head and back supported is supposed to relax the abdominal wall, however this position is not very comfortable for patients who have an abdominal incision or who have a very forward poking chin. Crook Half Lying is a more comfortable alternative

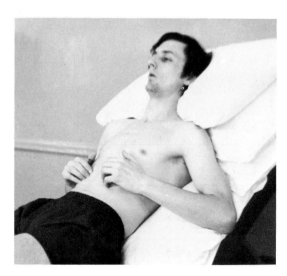

Figure 58 Half Lying practising diaphragmatic breathing.

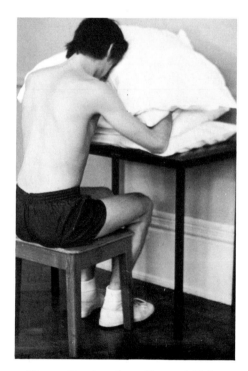

Figure 59 Arm Lean Forward Sitting.

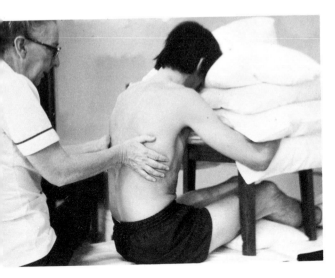

Figure 60 Arm Lean Forward Crook Sitting posterior basal breathing—therapist resisting.

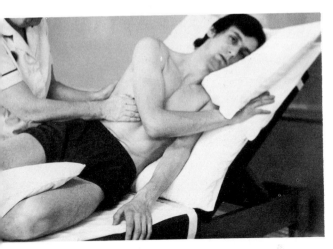

Figure 61 Half Side Lying.

for relieving tension of the abdominal muscles, but does not solve the problem of the kyphotic patient with a poking chin. Alternatives for such patients are Arm Lean Forward Sitting or Arm Lean Forward Crook Sitting. The patient will be placed at a table with a pile of pillows on which he rests his forearms at no more than shoulder height. One or two more pillows are placed on top of the forearms and the head rests on these (Figure 59). In Arm Lean Forward Crook Sitting the patient may rest his elbows on his knees and his head on his hands, or a pile of pillows is placed on his knees or on his bedtable and he is placed as above (Figure 60).

Another comfortable position is one of side support. This may be Side Lying, Side Half Lying (Figure 61) or Lean Side Standing. In the latter case the lower thorax should be slack or bent slightly to allow easier deep breathing.

Children will also use Kneel Sitting with the arms supported in the Forward Lean position or adults may use Relaxed Sitting with the elbows resting on the knees, Forward Lean Standing or Back Lean Standing when the hips and back are leant against a wall. In any of the above positions, any of the breathing exercises may be taught, provided the patient is relatively relaxed and has learnt basically to keep the shoulder girdle relaxed when it is not fully supported.

Therapist's position

The therapist may sit on the bed or be in Walk Standing leaning across the patient either from in front (facing) or from behind (facing his back). She should select her position to give even, maximum resistance or indication of respiratory movement, without allowing the patient to infect her and at the same time be able to observe or feel the chest movement.

Diaphragmatic breathing

Diaphragmatic breathing is the most common

form of breathing which has to be taught to a patient.

With the patient in a relaxed position, the therapist places the patient's finger tips or her own finger tips or the length of her thumbs along the costal margins and makes the patient aware of the 'boney' edges (Figure 59). The patient is then instructed to breathe out by asking him to '*blow gently*'. This will ensure an expiratory action and he is made aware of the inward movement of the costal margins. On the spontaneous breath in, which follows, the patient should be encouraged to try to move the costal margins further apart. If the diaphragm is being used in its middle–inner range the costal margins will separate, whereas the intercostal (central epigastric) area will swell slightly if the diaphragm is contracting in its outer range, i.e. the abdominal wall will bulge slightly.

As the patient becomes accustomed to this movement of the costal margins he should be asked to increase the distance of the movement—to take them nearer together on expiration and separate more widely on inspiration. As he does this the therapist should observe the whole chest to see that he is localizing his breathing to the lower part of the thorax at that time. If he starts to move the upper chest then he is using other muscles and is taking too deep a breath to maintain localization to diaphragmatic and lower thoracic expansion. Repeated practice should be encouraged in all the above positions until diaphragmatic breathing becomes spontaneous and natural.

Localized breathing

Localization of movement to any particular area of the thorax is possible with practice and the underlying lung tissue will probably expand more than any other part of the lung during that expansion. The skill is best practised against resistance. The patient is first suitably positioned, the therapist places her hand over the part to be exercised and the patient is instructed to '*blow*'. As he breathes out the therapist applies pressure to that part of the thorax increasing gradually as the patient reaches the limit of his movement of that part of the thorax. The therapist maintains her pressure as a resistance, telling the patient to breathe in '*under my hand*' and allowing the thorax to expand against her resistance which diminishes as the limit of the expansion is reached. This allows maximum expansion to occur. The hand positions are as follows:

Apical The fingers rest under the clavicle as flat as possible **or** the palms rest under the clavicle with the fingers held off the patient (Figure 62).

Lower lateral costal The hand rests with the little finger along the line of the eighth rib and

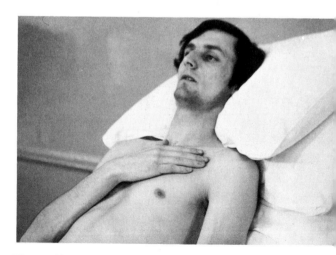

Figure 62 Apical breathing. Self resistance with the fingers.

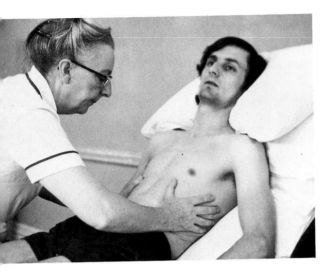

Figure 63   Lower lateral costal breathing—therapist resisting.

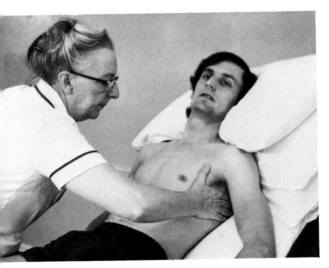

Figure 64   Upper lateral costal breathing—therapist resisting.

the whole hand in the obliquity of the ribs in mid-axillary area (Figure 63).

Upper lateral costal   Again in mid-axillary area,

the hands now less oblique, but still in line with the ribs, hand just under the axilla (Figure 64).

Posterior basal   The therapist sits on the bed behind the patient who leans forward and may be in Arm Lean Forward Sitting (Figure 60). The hands are placed fingers pointing out and down so that the heels of the hands rest just lateral to the rib angles. The hands lie along the line of the eighth, ninth, and tenth ribs, i.e. thumb just below the scapula in its normal resting position. The scapula may be protracted by the starting position. Very little movement may be felt here, yet training can produce satisfactory movement.

Self resistance

The patient may apply self resistance either with a flat hand, or, if his wrist extension is limited and he tends to hunch his shoulders, with the backs of his fingers (Figure 65).

He can do this for lower and upper lateral costal expansion using the hand of the same side, or the hand of the opposite side if he is to practise unilateral expansion. For apical breathing he *must* use the hand of the opposite side placing his fingers below the clavicle (Figure 62).

Use of a belt

A webbing strap about 5–10 cm wide may be found easier to use than the hand. It should be about 2 m long. It is wrapped round the lower chest and crossed in front, then the patient takes an overgrasp on the ends with his hands held pronated and between his hips and waist. On inspiration he resists his own movement by allowing the belt to slide slowly round his expanding thorax and on expiration slides the

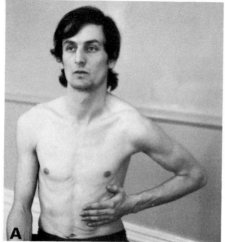

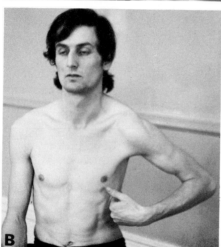

Figure 65 Self resistance unilateral **lower** costal breathing. A, With the whole hand; B, With the backs of the fingers.

two ends over one another to keep the belt in firm contact with the chest wall. If unilateral expansion is to be practised the patient sits and the lower crossed piece of the belt is tucked under the thigh and the upper crossed piece is held in the hand opposite to the side

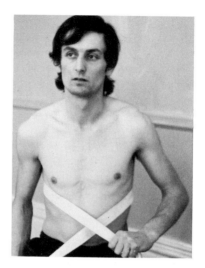

Figure 66 Using a belt for lower lateral costal breathing. The left hand is offering resistance to right sided expansion.

on which the chest is to be expanded (Figure 66).

Support for coughing

In general a most effective cough is obtained

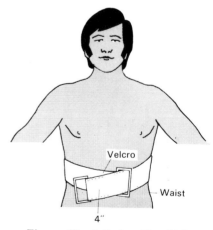

Figure 67 A Barlow Coughlok.

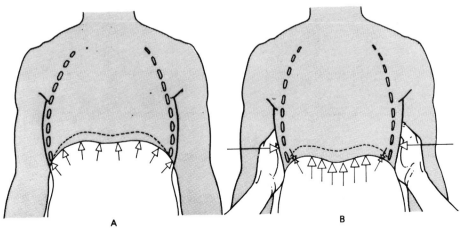

Figure 68 The diaphragm showing pressure exerted on it by a cough when the ribs are: A, unsupported; B, held firmly. B produces a more effective cough with less effort on the part of the patient.

when the abdominal wall is not on the stretch and these muscles can contract hard in their inner range. To effect this the hips should be bent, e.g. patient in Sitting or Crook Sitting and the back is slightly bent. The patient should try to take several deep breaths before attempting to cough, then breathe in, sharply contract the abdomen and cough (i.e. open the epiglottis) when ready. A more effective cough is brought about if the sides of the chest are held, either by the patient himself or the therapist using her hands in the line of the ribs again in mid axillary line; **or**, a webbing strap is held by the patient; **or**, a Barlow Coughlok is used which is a 20 cm wide strap with Velcro attached so that when the smaller metal loop is passed through the larger the Velcro engages and forms a firm belt to hold the chest wall (Figure 67).

In this way maximum use is made of the abdominal pressure upwards onto the thoracic contents instead of allowing some of the pressure to be dispersed sideways on to the lower and peripheral parts of the diaphragm (Figure 68).

Huffing

This is the term applied to a long, forceful expiration with the epiglottis open but without a cough.

The patient should be asked to take a big and deep (diaphragmatic) breath in, then to breathe out rapidly and powerfully making a strong 'sighing' sound. He should have relaxed lips and his mouth should be slightly open. The sound which emerges should come from his chest and not from his throat.

Alternatively, he may be asked to take a big breath in and then make a long, single cough. The sound at the end of this effort should be the 'huffing' sound. Thereafter he should be asked to 'huff' without coughing.

This action drives secretions up the respiratory tree so that they can be voided. The deeper the huff the more likely are deeply seated secretions to be driven towards the trachea. Each 'huff' is automatically accompanied by an abdominal contraction and relaxation of the diaphragm and patients who have difficulty with commanded breathing may find this action more automatic and therefore easier. A rest should be given after five or six attempts and asthmatic and dyspnoeic patients should alternate one 'huff' with one quiet relaxed breath in and out.

CHAPTER 8

Apparatus: Small and Large

M. HOLLIS & B. SANFORD

SMALL APPARATUS

Small apparatus may be used in as infinite a variety of ways as it exists and may be contained within a Physiotherapy Department. Basically three things may be done with any piece of small apparatus. One can 'get rid' of it, 'receive' it or 'hang on' to it. It is the permutations of these three factors with weight and size and material, their relationship to other people or objects, obstructions, distance and direction, that produces the variety of exercise.

Each piece of apparatus will also have two main uses. It may be used as an object to achieve a particular purpose, e.g. threading a needle with cotton, or it may be used for its innate properties. For example, most small pieces of apparatus may be pushed about and therefore may be a load and a means of obtaining the patient's interest to move an object from place to place. According to their innate properties some pieces of apparatus may be very resistant to being moved, while others may be moved very easily.

In the former case the movement of a heavy weight across a rough surface would form a resistance exercise, while rolling a ball across a smooth surface would give a speedy and therefore a mobilizing movement. Both would be a means of maintaining the patient's interest.

The properties of any piece of apparatus may also present disadvantages. Any apparatus of compressible material may be squeezed, but it must be the right size for the part which holds it, and if it is inelastic and therefore incapable of returning to its original shape after the squeeze, then further work will be involved in rearranging the apparatus. A piece of foam rubber if squeezed and released, compresses with the force, stores energy and returns to its original shape, a beanbag or sand inside a bag may be squeezed or pushed into a different shape, but no energy will be stored in this activity and the beans or sand will remain where they have been placed.

A ball may be bounced and will return if aimed properly but is of no use if the patient cannot change balance to catch it. Similarly a rubber quoit may be squeezed and thrown but unlike a ball will not return. A piece of material such as a band or pillowcase can be squeezed with little likelihood of it rolling or sliding away.

Some of the properties of some common pieces of small apparatus are discussed in the ensuing pages.

Whenever small apparatus is used it should have been experimented with by the therapist so that she is aware of the values and limitations which that object may have. Some apparatus is more useful for team games or where two patients are working together.

Experiments will also reveal that the method of use of each piece of apparatus will give a movement line or direction and weight. The weighting of the movement is dependent upon the energy which the patient imparts to the activity which he is trying to achieve. All movements are 'loaded' by the quality of the activity and in order to achieve greater or lesser loading by the patient he must be directed exactly as to the manner in which he should use the piece of apparatus with which he is practising. It is not necessary to use a heavy load, e.g. a 5 kg weight, to obtain strong extensor muscle work for the back muscles. Hard bouncing of a light ball against a wall through a long distance, especially a double-handed overhead throw, will work the back extensors very hard in inner range to prepare for the throw and in middle and inner range to catch a high returning ball.

In the same way the line or direction of a movement must be taught to the patient so that he moves the required joints. Whilst the therapist is placing her hands on the moving parts, direction and therefore line will be indicated, but free, objective and interesting movement may not achieve such perfection of line.

Initially perfection of line does not matter. The patient will achieve his objective the best way he can, constructive teaching and encouragement will improve the direction of the movement and adjustment of the starting position and method of performance will eventually improve the line and method of work.

Careful consideration has to be given at all times to the use of basic principles. The starting position should be selected to limit the movement to a particular part if the object is mainly to strengthen muscles locally or to limit movement to a small number of joints, but if strength and range are to be improved by corporate work of the whole body then a less limiting starting position should be chosen. Much will also depend on other factors and it is important to know if the patient is capable of static balance, has good dynamic balance, has good vision, cutaneous perception and coordination.

Safety of the patient using the apparatus and of other patients around should be considered. The load, whether in the form of weights or weighted balls, should be within his capacity. If he fetches equipment himself he will be revealed to be capable of doing this much with it. He should have the minimum equipment near him and apparatus should be moved to a safe place or put away in its storage place after use so that it does not constitute a hazard to other people in the vicinity.

The safety of the use of apparatus is dependent on the correct selection of a suitable piece of equipment for the task in hand. Injured elbows should not be treated by the use of weights or heavy balls, elderly people and small children need yielding pieces of apparatus so that if they miss a catch and are struck no damage is done. More agile patients can work with small rapidly moving pieces of equipment to which great energy may be imparted.

Finally, it should be observed by personal practice that by using apparatus it is not necessary to direct the patient's efforts all the time to the affected part of the body. Running bouncing a ball is as much an exercise for a weak or stiff foot, knee, hip, back, shoulder, elbow and hand as it is for poise, balance and coordination.

Balls

Balls may be used to exercise every part of the body by objective activity and the infinite variety of their size, weight and materials gives added value to their use.

One of the most important points to be considered before choosing to use a ball for any activity is the ability of the patient to retrieve it. The nature of a ball which is 'lost' by the patient is to continue its motion in the direction of the force last imparted to it and to continue until the energy is consumed or it meets an obstacle. A static patient who needs objective exercise should be given a non-rolling or less mobile object which he can retrieve if he misses or drops it.

If these properties are considered and related to the above three factors and to the three basic uses of apparatus ('hang on' to it, 'get rid' of it or 'receive' it) then some uses will emerge.

Balls may be solid such as a small ball bearing or marble used for fine intrinsic movements of the fingers, semi-solid such as a medicine ball made of a leather case and packing to a specific weight, or semi-solid but aerated in varying materials from sorbo rubber, the common ball of our youth, or from man-made materials varying in density and aeration from the Supa ball, which is small and needs little energy imparted to it to create bounce, to the polyurethane foam balls which are compressible round soft 'shapes'.

Aeration may be total, i.e. the ball is a case around a permanent supply of air, and the degree of bounce will depend on the air pressure inside the case. These balls need constant attention to their pressure and the larger balls may need to have air pumped into them regularly to make them harder and better bouncers. In time the casing will deteriorate with use and the ball will then need replacement as a bouncer but may still be used for its compressibility.

The size of ball matters in relation to the capacity of the patient as well as to the part to be exercised. Large and brightly coloured balls are best used for the very young and more elderly as the eye and body coordination demanded are least with such balls and at their maximum with small, 'fast', balls. (Some balls of artificial material have higher elastic properties and produce 'fast' response to a small force, e.g. Supa balls.)

The part of the body to catch, hold or retrieve the ball will also control the size of ball to be chosen. A hand with small span, i.e. which cannot be opened into full extension, needs a small ball, as a big ball demands full extension of the hand joints if it is to be held or caught. Fine foot movements can be performed using a small ball, but most people need a bigger ball for coarse foot movements or leg movements. On the whole a large ball is easier to control, but may require fuller range movements if it is to be held.

The distance through which a ball is thrown will alter both the joints moved and the muscles worked. Try the following experiment:

Take a small hand-held sorbo rubber ball. Stand near to a wall on to which it can be thrown and have a clear space behind you. Start throwing the ball overarm and one handed at the wall and walk backwards a half pace between each throw. Get a colleague to observe your movements and think about your own muscle work. Near to the wall the head and neck must be extended as well as having the arm elevated and elbow extended to perform the throw. As the distance from the wall increases the head and neck movement is lost and the whole arm is flexed and extended, then the upper trunk is rotated and finally the legs are flexed and extended to impart thrust to the ball.

Repeat the same activities with an underarm throw and then with a double-handed throw, both under- and overarm, and observe which position produces most movement and therefore most muscle work for each part of the body. Some of the positions and types of throw are obviously more mobilizing. That is, they carry the body component past a potentially blocked point in the range. In the case of other positions and types of throw the effect is more one of strengthening for various muscle groups. That is, the amount of effort imparted to the ball is greater and therefore the muscles work harder.

Now continue to explore the uses of the different sizes, weights, and types of balls, using ball and floor, ball and wall, ball and air space, ball and body relationships in, say, Standing, Sitting and Lying using the ball with the upper limb/s for finger and thumb, hand, wrist, radio-ulnar, elbow and shoulder movements; with the lower limb/s for toe, foot, ankle, knee and hip movements. Consider which, if any, of these involve the trunk and/or head to enhance the movement, increase the muscle effort or ensure coordination.

Do not forget that a ball can be kicked, kneed, hipped, shouldered or headed if it is suitable and the action appropriate to the needs of the patient. Also discover that space may control selection of the ball size and weight. To throw a light ball in such a way that movement of the lower thoracic or lumbar spine is produced needs a long space. The same effect will be produced in less than half the space if a 1 kg medicine ball is substituted with no very great increase in effort for the trunk muscles, but considerably more effort for the arm muscles.

The way in which a ball is held in the hand will also produce variations in joints used and muscles worked. The type of grip must be adapted to the size and weight of the ball and so must the manner in which the ball is to be thrown or received, e.g. overarm, underarm, single handed or double handed.

Quoits

These are rings of about 20 cm (8 in) diameter made of either sorbo rubber or rope. If the former they have the property of elasticity, if the latter they will be semi-rigid.

Only the sorbo rubber quoit can be turned inside out involving movement of all the upper limb joints and work of mucles against resistance, but both types offer other similar features.

They form a ring round a space and so can be used for all threading activities whether it be transfer from foot to foot, passing a stick or hand through them or 'aiming' to thread or throw them over a skittle or hand-held pole.

They are a circle of material and can be gripped by foot or hand by one person or by two people and so used for pushing, pulling and twisting exercises, done in Standing, Sitting or Long Sitting.

A quoit is also a suitable object to be rolled or thrown though the rope quoits will roll less well than the rubber quoits and both types are objects which may be pushed over higher structures such as the top of the wall bars or thrown to a partner over a beam or high rope. A quoit may also be tied on the end of a rope as a weight so that it can be whipped in a circle and jumped over in leg exercises thus increasing timing ability in eye and leg coordination.

A quoit is sometimes substituted for a ball in games such as deck tennis when the space is confined. It is of value in such games because it rolls less if the receiver fails to catch it and therefore requires movement through only short distances in order to retrieve it.

Hoops

Hoops may be made of bamboo or other wood and may be somewhat uneven and brittle, or of plastic and therefore even, but compressible. They are of varying sizes and may be of small enough diameter to be used to pass the body through in 'mock dressing', or of large enough diameter to be run through as the hoop bowls along.

Spinning a hoop (hula-hoop) may be done with the whole body, any part of the upper or lower limb and in so doing, very complex movements will be performed in a coordinated manner. Alternatively a hoop can be rotated between hand and the ground or a wall, so producing finely coordinated finger and thumb movements with the arm in many different relationships to the trunk while dynamic balance is maintained.

A hoop may be used as a fixed outline enclosing a space enabling many jumping, stepping, bouncing games to be devised, or the outline may be used for coordinated leg movements by stepping round the margin of the hoop.

Suspended hoops can form part of an obstacle course and can be held by a partner as a stepping or jumping obstacle.

Ropes

Many activities with a rope involve the use of the hands and arms. Ropes can be of a length of about 2 m for individual use or of any longer length to allow group participation. They should preferably be made of hemp and can vary in diameter from approximately 1·5 cm to many centimetres, when weight will become a feature to be considered. On the whole lighter weight ropes are usually used for individual work but a heavier texture is more useful and 'whips' and deviates less than the light rope and thus is more useful for group work.

Ropes for individual use are more useful if the ends are bound and sealed, and not fixed to handles.

The most obvious use of a rope is for various forms of skipping and jumping exercises performed either slowly or quickly, thus involving arm and leg movement and great coordination.

But a rope can be used for intrinsic work with the hands, when one or both is incoordinate. It may be tied into a malleable circle and used as though dressing and it can be laid on the ground and stepped along in a straight or wriggling path.

The whole length of the rope can be crumpled by hand or feet and if bound together it becomes a non-bouncing object which may be used for target work.

With a quoit tied to one end and the therapist or a patient holding the other end the rope may be swung round in circles while the remaining patients forming a ring jump over it as it passes. If a patient is swinging the rope he can sit or stand according to his ability. He might even be a patient with a disablement of the shoulder or arm and so work with patients who need primarily leg exercises.

A rope may also be used to create shapes on the floor and to be an obstacle to be jumped over, climbed up or pulled as in a tug-of-war.

Bands

These are soft webbing or braid in a variety of colours and of a length of approximately

75–100 cm, sewn at the ends to make a circular band. Like a rope their uses are multiple.

First, as they are flat and of moderately rough material they have a high coefficient of friction, they will therefore stay where they are dropped, put down or tucked in. They can, in consequence, be used as markers of all sorts, either as a tail in chasing games, a marker on a rope for tug-of-war, or for distance jumped or hopped.

The material is just springy enough to be a challenge in pulling the whole length of the band into the hand or under the foot by lumbrical action or by digital flexion, which-ever is desired.

Since the bands are soft and tend to cling they can be used for dressing and undressing practice before a patient is ready to tackle putting on or taking off actual clothing.

A series of bands looped into one another will make an emergency rope of some length and they can be looped round hoops or quoits as a means of hanging these objects up. A series of experiments on the lines suggested for balls will reveal that they can be used in a similar manner but as non-returning objects, and their use need not be limited to marking the members of the red and blue teams.

Beanbags

A beanbag is usually made of cotton twill squares so that a flat bag approximately 20–30 cm square is produced containing enough dried beans to half fill the bag. It should be double stitched at all seams.

This produces a small object of variable shape and with no elastic properties. If thrown it must land and be fetched or be caught and returned. It can thus be used for aiming or target exercises with or without a partner.

Without a partner the target can be a bucket, bowl, hoop, rope or band circle and the patient will need quite a pile of beanbags to keep him busy. Additional exercise is provided by the initial positioning of the stock of beanbags. Thus a sitting patient may have to pick up his beanbag from his right with his right hand and so side flex, and/or flex and/or extend according to where on his right the beanbags are placed. Alternatively, they may be put on his left and he must then rotate and flex or extend and perhaps also extend his left arm for propping purposes. The object of the exercise might then well be to use the left arm for this purpose and recover balance after the target practice.

Many finger and hand exercises can be performed with beanbags as they may be used above or on a table. Each bean may be mani-pulated across the bag and stereognostic ability increased, or the bag may be flicked with flexion, extension, ulnar or radial deviation of the wrist or with any of the movements of the fingers and thumb. The smaller bags are especially useful for flicking exercises where rapid digital extension must be performed.

As they are a handsized object to grip they can simulate a duster, wash leather or dish-cloth for domestic tasks and so be a means of performing unloaded arm, leg and trunk movements in full range and in a functional way.

Poles

Wooden rods of varying lengths and diameters and thus of varying weights provide a means of devising a challenging variety of exercises.

A thin pole such as a broomstick handle is approximately 1250 cm long and 2 cm in diameter whereas a pole which is the same diameter as a tennis ball, i.e. functional grip size, may be 10–15 cm in diameter and would be very heavy if it were 1250 cm long. However, such a pole would still have its uses in heavy resistance exercise and for those without fine grip.

Most exercises using poles involve the hand and arm directly as grip is usually needed. Exceptions are paired exercises in which a thicker pole is placed on the floor between two people each in Crook Sitting with their heels on the floor on the far side of the pole from themselves. They try to pull the pole with their heels thus flexing the hips and knees and working the hamstrings hard. Or the pole may be used as a 'raise' over which to exercise the foot lumbricals or be rolled (underfoot) in Sitting moving the foot through dorsi- and plantarflexion and the knee in middle range.

The trunk muscles and leg muscles are mainly exercised by again either using pairs of people to twist, pull up and down or side to side on a suitable pole or by passing people in a circle round a series of standing poles in a ring. The idea being speedy leg, trunk and arm movement to catch each pole while it is still vertical.

Solo exercises might involve pronation and supination using a grip at the middle of the pole and the long weight arm on each side as the load. Rolling out pastry across a table, rolling a pole up the wall are progressively harder arm exercises, or again it may be an object to be jumped over, walked round or stepped over. Its advantage in these cases is its mobility in one plane by rolling which is also its disadvantage. That is, if the patient lands on the pole it will roll under his foot and he will initially need the therapist on hand as a 'catcher' until his balance is sound.

LARGE APPARATUS

Large apparatus can be space-consuming and good organization is necessary for its use. Patients who are moving it should constantly be aware of its potential danger to others in the room, e.g. when lowering a beam, although the patient's body will face the controlling rope, the face should be turned to look at the centre of the room ready to react to prevent other patients being hit on the head.

Wallbars

These may be fixed permanently to the wall or on hinges which allow them to be turned at an angle to the wall. In this position both sides can be used and they provide a climbing frame for suitable groups. Other uses are listed below.

1 As a support for a patient's back
2 As a hand support to aid balance or to gain height in upward jumps
3 As a target for progressive upward stepping and jumping or for tying and aiming objects and for touching
4 For progressing height in landing training
5 For heaving and grasping exercises
6 As a support for other apparatus
7 As an attachment for pulley systems and springs

Forms

These can be used with either the broad or narrow side uppermost. Patients should avoid stepping on the upturned feet as this will cause the form to tip sideways and throw them off. They have many different uses.

1 For retraining balance especially in weight-bearing positions
2 As a target for jumping over
3 As a platform for stepping and jumping on to and off
4 To simulate a step or an incline
5 As a low seat
6 As an object for lifting (always use two people)
7 As a low target for aiming at or over
8 As an area divider

Beams

These can be very dangerous if they are incorrectly fixed for use and the therapist should check before allowing patients to work on them. The wedges should be inserted at each end of the beam and from above, only if this is upturned for balance work as they stop a perpetual sideways movement. Their uses are:

1 For heaving exercises with the body suspended or supported
2 As a target for stepping over, under or between
3 As a target for crawling or wriggling under
4 As a target for aiming purposes and for touching whilst continuing to move forward
5 As a means of fixation for suspension and pulleys
6 As a support for other apparatus, e.g. saddles or forms
7 As a hand support at variable heights
8 Used upside down for balance exercises

Vaulting apparatus (box, horse and buck)

These are mainly used for advanced agility work. Patients who are returning to jobs or hobbies demanding quick or slow controlled coordinated movements of the whole body will benefit from performing the standard vaults. Details of these can be found in specialist books on the subject. This apparatus can also be used to provide a high, firm, wide base for the hands for weightbearing exercises for the upper limbs. The box particularly can be used as a wide platform for training mounting and dismounting using both hands and feet.

Prevention of accidents in vaulting

The therapist should always position herself close to the apparatus on the side where the patient will land. This will give him confidence to attack the vault. She should stand with her feet apart and positioned so that she can transfer her weight from one foot to the other in the direction of the movement of the vaulter without overbalancing. She can then safely intervene if an accident looks imminent, but need not interfere with the free movement of a well executed vault. To support the patient, the therapist should use her offside shoulder to block his body and grasp with both hands round his nearside upper arm. She should *never* place her hands on either side of his elbow joint as this often leads to injury. All patients using vaulting apparatus should have full knowledge of the principles of landing.

Trampolines

These are available in various sizes. The small ones are often used to give extra spring and body propulsion to enable less advanced patients to gain satisfactory elevation when first attempting to use the vaulting apparatus. The larger trampolines need specialist skills and activities on these should only be taught by therapists with extensive experience of their use.

Climbing ropes

Movement of ropes must be carefully controlled as they swing dangerously when moved quickly. The controlling pulley rope must be firmly anchored round the wall hook to ensure correct spacing between the ropes and prevent body contact when more than one person is using them. They are used for exercises in which the body weight is supported on the arms or legs.

They can be climbed either singly or in pairs. If two are used the feet should grasp both ropes together and the hands should grasp each rope separately. The latter method allows a better position of the shoulders, but the footgrasp is more difficult to hold. Patients may transfer sideways from rope to rope or climb diagonally upwards or downwards as the transfer is made.

Swinging is possible using either one rope or two, and by grasping with the hands only or with both feet and hands if only one rope is used. They can maintain their own propulsion by bending and then extending the knees strongly pushing the feet out in the direction of the movement, or by a few running steps in either direction at the points when the feet can reach the ground if two ropes are used. If necessary, the therapist can maintain the swing by gently pushing the patient's bottom. Ropes can also be used for hanging upside down. If two ropes are used a complete somersault either forwards or backwards may be executed.

Patients should come down ropes hand over hand as sliding quickly may cause friction burns to the hands and to that part of the legs in contact with the ropes whether or not it is protected by clothing.

CHAPTER 9
Suspension

M. HOLLIS

Suspension is the means whereby parts of the body are supported in slings and elevated by the use of variable length ropes fixed to a point above the body. Suspension frees the body from the friction of the material upon which body components may be resting and it permits free movement without resistance when the fixation is suitably arranged relative to the supported part.

All that is needed for suspension to be effected is a fixed point (hook) above the relevant part of the body and a Suspensory Unit which consists of a sling and an adjustable rope (Figure 69).

The fixed point

It is common present-day practice to fit stainless steel or plastic covered metal mesh of a 5 cm mesh and of suitable total sizes to cover the area of a plinth, i.e. 1 m or 2 m wide × 2 m long above and perhaps on the wall at the side of the plinth 2 m × 2 m and at the head of the plinth 1 m or 2 m × 2 m long and 2 m high (Figure 70).

It is usual to suspend the overhead mesh from the ceiling joists at a height which will allow about 1·5 m clearance between mesh and plinth top.

If it is impossible to fix mesh on to the ceiling because of the nature of the ceiling structure then a free-standing frame may be used

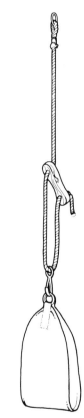

Figure 69 A suspensory unit consisting of a rope and a sling.

(Figure 71). This is a frame big enough to take a single bed, i.e. 2 m long × 1 m wide at the base and a somewhat narrower top

68

frame which is serrated on the upper surface of both the frame and linking bars. Hooks on the side of the frame allow lateral fixed points and can be used to keep the small apparatus near at hand.

Storage

Storage of slings and ropes can otherwise be on a wall frame of suitable hooks or on a mobile trolley as in Figure 72. Hooks with a large and small curve are used (Figure 73).

The supporting ropes

Ropes should be of 3-ply hemp so that they will not slip and may be of three arrangements.

Single rope

This has a ring fixed at one end by which it is hung up. The other end of the rope then passes through one end of a wooden cleat, through the ring of a dog clip and through the other end of the cleat (Figure 69) and is then knotted with a half-hitch. The cleat is for altering the length of the rope and should be held horizontally for movement and pulled oblique when supporting (Figure 74). The rope then 'holds' on the cleat by frictional resistance. The dog clip should be on a pivot to allow adjustments in position with minimum discomfort when the slings are attached. The total length of rope required is 1·5 m.

Further shortening of the rope may be brought about by knotting it about the cleat, as in Figure 75, so that the supporting end is

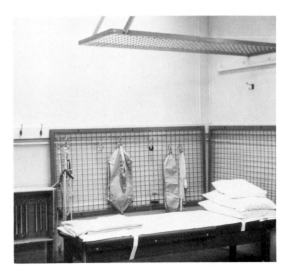

Figure 70 A mesh arrangement to cover a large area and allow many variations in 'fixed points'.

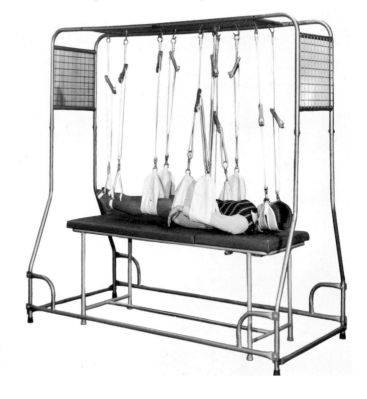

Figure 71 A free-standing frame designed by the late Mrs Guthrie Smith MBE. The suspension is vertical for all body parts.

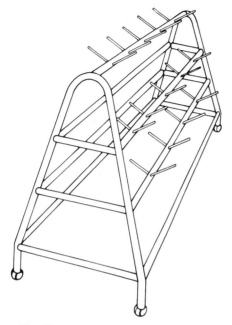

Figure 72 One aspect only of an original design of a trolley to accommodate all the suspension equipment, pulleys, springs and handles needed for a large hospital. The trolley is shown minus equipment for clarity. Both sides have hooks for equipment and the hooks are arranged to allow the equipment to hang inside the castors and base frame.

firm, but the free end can be pulled out and permanent knots are not made.

Pulley rope

This has a dog clip attached to one end of the rope which then passes over the wheel of a pulley. The rope then passes through the cleat and a second dog clip as described above (Figure 76). This rope is also 1·5 m long. This arrangement is used for reciprocal pulley circuits, and with one sling supporting a limb the ends of which are attached to the two dog clips it is used for three-dimensional movements of a limb, i.e. abduction or adduction

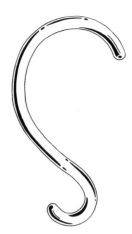

Figure 73 An 'S' hook which may be used either end according to the size of the 'fixed point'.

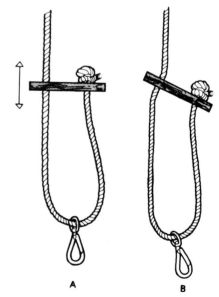

Figure 74 A, The cleat in the horizontal position for changing the length of the rope; B, The cleat in the oblique position in which frictional resistance causes it to 'hold' its own position.

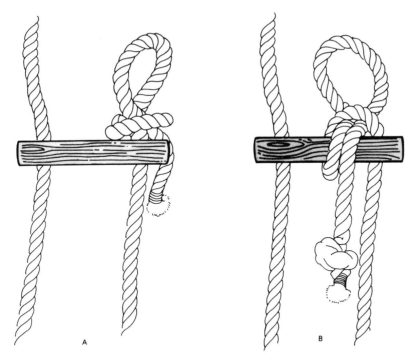

Figure 75 Two alternative methods (A and B) of shortening a rope with the free end held in such a manner that a tug on it enables quick release.

with flexion or extension and medial or lateral rotation (combined, oblique, rotatory movements).

Double rope

This consists of a ring and clip at the upper end by which the rope can be hung up which creates a compensating device to permit a certain amount of swivel on the rope. The rope then passes through one side of a cleat, round a pulley wheel at the lower end of the rope to the case of which is attached a dog clip, through the other end of the cleat, over the wheel of an upper pulley which is attached to the compensating device. The rope then passes down again through a centre hole in the cleat where it is knotted (Figure 77). This device gives a mechanical advantage of two, as two pulleys are used. The rope is shortened by pushing the cleat down, allowing the lifter to move with gravity at the same time as it offers a mechanical advantage of two. Such a rope is used to suspend the heavy parts of the body—the pelvis, thorax or heavy thighs when these are to be supported together.

Slings

Single slings are made of canvas bound with soft webbing and with a D ring at each end (Figure 78,A). They are used open to support the limbs or folded in two and as a figure of eight to support the hand or foot (Figures

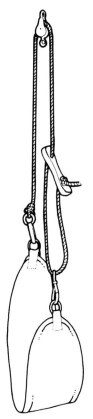

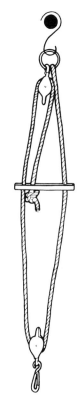

Figure 76 A pulley rope—used for auto-pulley circuits or to allow rotation combined with angular movements.

Figure 77 A double pulley rope having a mechanical advantage of two.

79,A,B and 80,A). They measure 68 cm long by 17 cm wide.

Double slings are broad slings measuring 68 cm long by 29 cm wide with D rings at each end and are used to support the pelvis or thorax or the thigh together, especially when the knees are to be kept straight (Figure 78,B).

Three-ring slings These are webbing slings 71 cm long by 3–4 cm wide with three D rings, one fastened at each end and one free in the

middle. The centre ring is for attachment to the dog clip and the webbing is slipped through the end D rings to make two loops (Figure 78,D,E). These slings are used to support the wrist and hand or ankle and foot (Figures 79,C and 80,B).

Head sling This is a short, split sling with its two halves stitched together at an angle to create a central slit. This allows the head to rest supported at the back under the lower and upper parts of the skull, or in the Side Lying position leaves the ear free. Skilful tilting of the sling when it is applied in Side Lying will

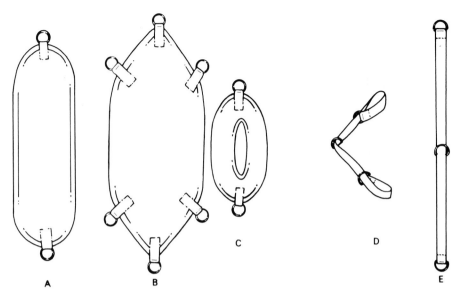

Figure 78 A, A single sling; B, A double sling; C, A head sling; D, A three-ring sling ready for use; E, A three-ring sling ready for storage.

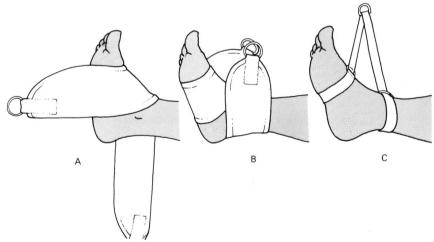

Figure 79 A and B, A single sling folded and being made into a figure of eight for use on the foot and ankle; C, A three-ring sling on the foot and ankle.

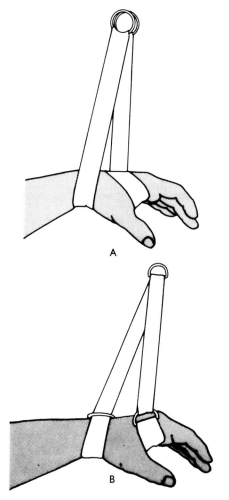

Figure 80   A, The single sling folded for use as a figure of eight on the hand; B, The three-ring sling on the hand.

arrange it so that the front ring lies at the level of the forehead and not over the eyes and nose, the other half lies below the occiput (Figure 78,C).

Clips   Carabine hooks (Figure 81,B) of 70 mm or 100 mm now provide a convenient alter-

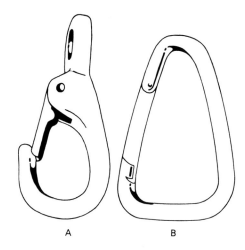

Figure 81   A, A dog clip; B, A carabine clip.

native means of clipping two pieces of equipment together.

TYPES OF SUSPENSION

Vertical fixation

In using this fixation the rope is fixed so that it hangs vertically above the centre of gravity of the part to be suspended. The centre of gravity of each part of the body is, on the whole, at the junction of the upper and middle one-third (Figure 5, p. 11). Vertical suspension is used for support as it will be found that it tends to limit the movement of the part to a small-range pendular movement on each side of the central resting point (Figure 82,A,B). It is advisable to carry out an experiment suspending the lower limb, for example, from two points, the leg from above the tibia and the thigh from above the femur and then to attempt movement. It will be noted that the leg rises on each side in the lower sling and as it does so the thigh leaves the support of the

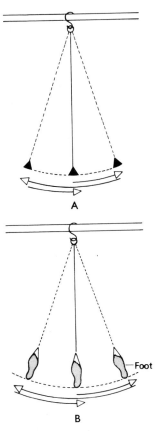

Figure 82 A, A pendulum; B, The foot, supported at the centre of gravity of the leg, acts like a pendulum.

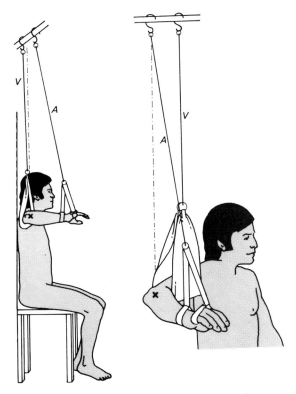

Figure 83 Vertical fixation by rope *V* for the arm. Axial fixation by rope *A* for the forearm. · – · · – · is the axis from the suspension point of rope *A* immediately above the elbow joint (×).

upper sling. In other words, the support is partly lost and the movement is limited by the length of the ropes. Vertical fixation is used primarily to support, e.g. the abducted upper limb when the elbow is to be moved is supported from above the centre of gravity of the arm and axial fixation is used over the elbow for the forearm (Figure 83).

Axial fixation

This occurs when all the ropes supporting a part are attached to one 'S' hook which is fixed to a point immediately above the centre of the joint which is to be moved, e.g. if the lower limb is to be moved at the hip joint two ropes, one to the foot and one to the area of the knee, will be used and fixed at a point immediately over the axis of the hip joint (Figure 84,B). When such fixation is set up the movement of the limb will be on a flat plane level with the floor. In this way pure angular movements are obtained (Figure 84,A).

If some resistance to the muscle work is

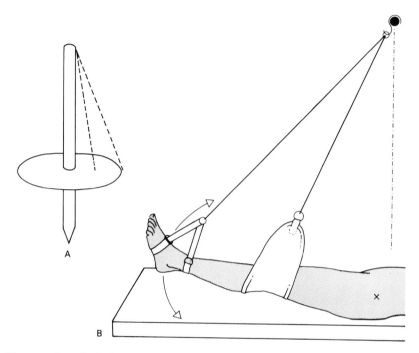

Figure 84 A, The pencil pushed through a circle of paper demonstrates that when the pencil is pivoted the paper moves in a plane parallel with the floor, thus demonstrating the principle of axial fixation; B, Axial fixation for adduction and abduction of the hip (– · – · – axial line, × hip joint).

required then the whole fixed point is moved away from the muscles which require resistance. If abduction is to be resisted the fixed point is moved towards the adductors and the limb then falls towards that side, i.e. into adduction. On effort the limb will now rise into abduction brought about by isotonic shortening of the abductors, resistance being offered by gravity. Slow lowering into the resting position is controlled by isotonic lengthening of the abductors, the movement is assisted by the pull of gravity and if, at any time, the abductors relax, the leg will drop into adduction. Figure 85 shows the method of finding the centre of gravity (A) and the axis (B).

Suspension for the lower extremity
The hip

Abduction and adduction The starting position is Lying with the opposite leg abducted to its limit even if the knee has to be bent over the side of the plinth and the foot supported on a footstool. The fixation point is immediately above the hip joint. One sling is put under the lower thigh and one three-ring sling on the foot and ankle and each is attached to a rope

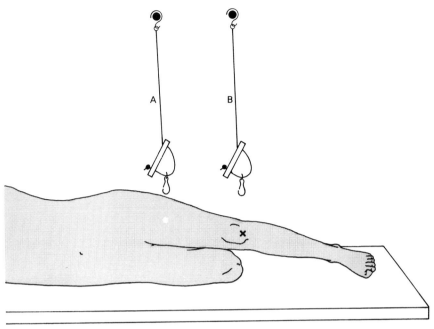

Figure 85   Rope A, suspended over the centre of gravity of the thigh. Rope B, suspended over the axis of the knee joint and ready to support the leg and foot.

hung from the fixation point. The limb is lifted just clear of the plinth. Using this method of support the movements of abduction and adduction may be mobilized or the abductor or adductor muscles may be especially worked with or without manual resistance (Figure 86).

Flexion and extension   The starting position is Side Lying with the underneath leg flexed as far as possible. The fixation point and sling arrangements are as above with the limb lifted until it is horizontal. If the movement of flexion is to be mobilized the knee and hip must be flexed together to overcome the passive insufficiency of the hamstrings. Equally, when mobilizing extension the knee should be extended to overcome active insufficiency of the hamstrings (Figure 87).

The knee

Flexion and extension   The starting position is Side Lying with one or two pillows between the slightly flexed thighs. One three-ring sling is applied to the foot and ankle and one rope attached to a fixation point above the knee joint. By keeping the hip slightly flexed on the trunk the foot can be seen each time the knee is extended and part of the arc of movement is thus observed by the patient. This position may be used to mobilize the knee joint or to work the flexors or extensors of the knee (Figure 88).

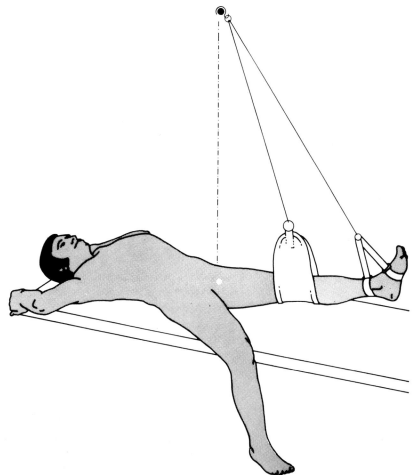

Figure 86　Abduction and adduction of the hip joint in axial fixation (− · − · − axial line).

The ankle

It is rarely necessary to use suspension as in this case it is easier to perform supported movements by using a polished board.

Suspension for the upper extremity

The shoulder joint

Abduction and adduction　The starting position is Lying, quarter turned towards the arm which is to be moved (Figure 89,A). This allows the normal anatomical movement to be performed in the plane of the scapula. *Alternatively*, Prone Lying, quarter turned towards Side Lying with a pillow under the trunk on the side of the arm which is to be moved (Figure 89,B). The advantage of Prone Lying is that the therapist can see the movements

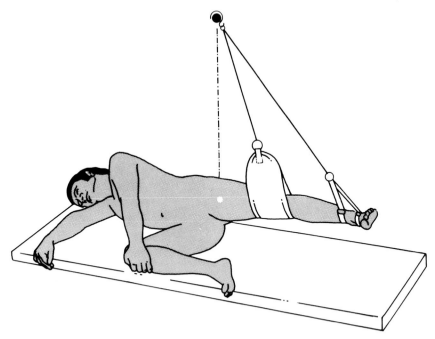

Figure 87 Flexion and extension of the hip joint in axial fixation (– · – · – axial line).

of the scapula as well as those of the arm.

Two single ropes are required. One attached to a single sling under the elbow and one to a three-ring sling applied to the wrist and hand. The fixation point is over the shoulder joint.

If the movement is to be only of the glenohumeral joint then the therapist must stand on the opposite side with one hand on the point of the shoulder depressing the scapula. In this form of support either abduction and adduction of the glenohumeral joint or movements of the shoulder girdle may be mobilized. Glenohumeral rhythm may be re-educated and all the muscles performing shoulder girdle movements may be worked.

Flexion and extension The starting position is Side Lying on pillows and quarter turned to the back. Female patients need two pillows under the head and one under the shoulder to allow the forearm to clear their wider pelvis.

The slings and ropes are arranged as described above and again the movement may be limited to the glenohumeral joint and the muscles working over it or movements of the shoulder girdle may be included.

If in addition to the angular movements it is desired to perform rotation of the glenohumeral joint then only one sling should be used at the level of the elbow and a single pulley rope attached to the fixed point above the shoulder. The ends of the sling are attached to each end of the pulley circuit and it will then be possible to perform medial or lateral rotation with two angular movements (Figures 90 and 91).

It will be necessary to turn the patient further towards the side or more prone. It is

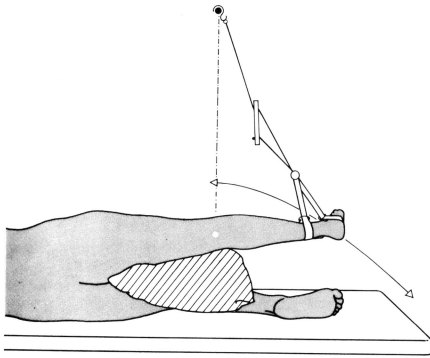

Figure 88   A pillow is placed between the thighs for flexion and extension of the knee in axial fixation (– · – · – axial line).

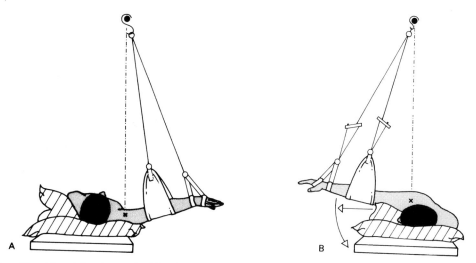

Figure 89   Shoulder abduction and adduction in axial fixation. A, Quarter 15° turned from Lying; B, Quarter 15° turned from Prone Lying. This position may also be used for protraction and retraction of the scapula (– · – · – axial line).

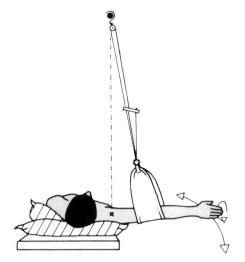

Figure 90 Using axial fixation over the right gleno-humeral joint and a single pulley rope the movements of extension/adduction/medial rotation and flexion/abduction/lateral rotation can be performed with the patient quarter 15° turned to the right (—·—·— axial line).

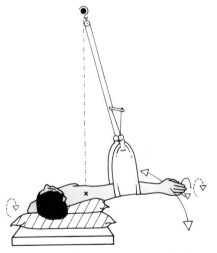

Figure 91 Using axial fixation over the right gleno-humeral joint and a single pulley rope the movements of extension/abduction/medial rotation and flexion/adduction/lateral rotation can be performed with the patient quarter 15° turned to the left (—·—·— axial line).

then possible to perform flexion, adduction and lateral rotation alternately with extension, abduction and medial rotation or flexion, abduction and lateral rotation alternately with extension, adduction and medial rotation.

Elbow joint

Flexion and extension Because of the carrying angle of the forearm it is easier to perform these movements when the arm is suspended in abduction. The starting position is Sitting on a low-backed chair. A single sling and rope supports the arm in vertical fixation and a three-ring sling and single rope are fixed to a point above the elbow joint (Figure 83). The therapist should stand behind as she may need to give additional support by holding the arm with a grasp inside the sling which will allow palpation of the flexors and extensors which are covered by the supporting sling. Alternatively, a folded single sling under the palm attached to a single pulley rope will allow pronation and supination to occur with extension and flexion of the elbow joint.

Wrist

Flexion and extension This is more usually and conveniently performed on a polished board or table.

Flexion and extension of the whole arm

As a functional movement this may be performed with the patient in the Sitting position, i.e. practising taking the hand to the mouth may be done by using two single slings attached to two single pulley rope circuits. One sling is placed round the arm and one round the forearm. If the ropes are sufficiently tightened the patient can grasp, supinate and flex the elbow and shoulder while adducting and laterally rotating. This sort of support is used for patients who have difficulty in performing personal facial toilet, feeding, turning the pages of a book fixed at eye level, or working in front of themselves.

Suspension for the trunk

It is more usual to perform trunk movement by suspending the pelvis and lower extremities as they provide a longer weight arm which can be varied in length by bending the knees, and it is easier for the patient to use his arms to help to fix the upper half of the body.

The starting position is a Low Half Lying

for side flexion and Side Lying for flexion and extension.

The fixed point has to be linear as it is not easily possible to put all the ropes on one hook. The line of hooks should be across the level of the third lumbar vertebra (umbilical line).

The following ropes and slings will be needed:

Two double ropes to each side of a large sling under the pelvis and fastened to the outer ends of the line of hooks.

Two single ropes to a sling supporting the thighs and on two hooks inside the pelvic supports.

One single rope to two three-ring slings,

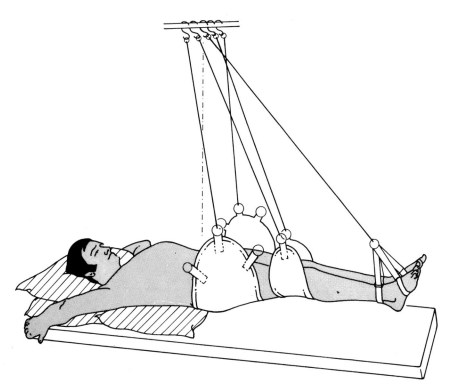

Figure 92   Heave Grasp Half Lying trunk side flexion using a linear axis over the level of L.3 (–·–·– axial line).

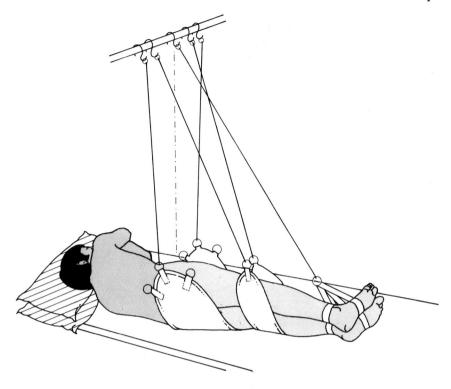

Figure 93 Forward Grasp Side Lying trunk flexion and extension using a linear axis over the level of L.3 (–·–·– axial line).

one on each foot and ankle and fastened at the top to the central hook. This rope keeps the feet fastened together and makes the lower extremities move as one unit. In Side Lying one foot will fall slightly in front of the other which prevents the medial malleoli from rubbing on each other.

For side flexion The patient holds in a Heave Grasp position and the ropes are shortened, knees, feet, pelvis in that order so that the body is just clear of the support and the knees are slightly flexed (Figure 92).

Enormous momentum can be built up in free swinging, and good mobilization can be obtained. To offer resistance to the muscles the therapist half kneels level with the lower thorax and grasps at the level of the waist on the opposite side. She offers resistance with the more distal hand either on the lower limb or on the thigh rope or sling. In this way right and left side flexors may be worked in full or part range in isotonic shortening or lengthening.

For flexion and extension The patient holds in Forward Heave Grasp (Figure 93) and the ropes are shortened until the legs are straight and the pelvis is just clear of the plinth. If flexion is the desired movement the thigh and

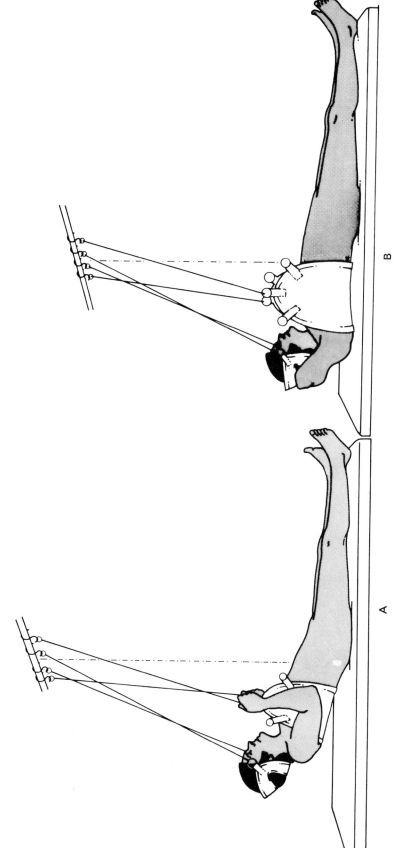

Figure 94 Alternative positions (A and B) for the arms for trunk side flexion by moving the head and thorax (—·—·— axial line).

foot ropes are moved to be fixed lateral to the front pelvic rope and the knees should be kept straight to limit hip movement by the passive insufficiency from the hamstrings. If extension is the desired movement then the thigh and foot ropes are moved to outside the rear pelvic rope and the knees are allowed to bend slightly on extension of the trunk to limit hip extension.

More commonly a combined knee, hip and trunk movement is practised with flexion or extension of all joints together and again great momentum can be built up. In this case the ropes are fixed as for side flexion. Resisted work may be given to the straight flexors and extensors by kneeling as described above and

offering resistance on a convenient part of the lower limb or on the thigh rope.

If for any reason it is necessary to move the upper trunk then it will be necessary to support the head separately and the upper extremities either by crossing them on the chest or separately supporting them in arm slings.

The head is supported on a head sling from two single ropes fixed at the level of the manubriosternal junction to allow the head to be raised and held in normal flexion.

The thorax is supported on a large sling by means of two double-pulley ropes and if the arms are supported separately they are held in a single sling each above the level of the elbow

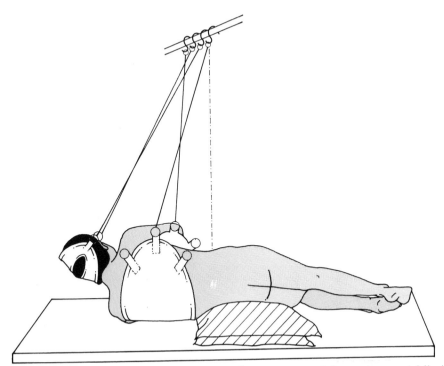

Figure 95 Trunk flexion and extension by moving the head and thorax (–·–·– axial line).

to two ropes each attached outside the thorax ropes. The forearms are then usually bent so that a grasp is taken on the sling. Some patients prefer to do without the arm slings and ropes and just to hold on to the double-pulley ropes (Figures 94 and 95).

It will be found that flexion and extension and side flexion are more limited in this form of support, but it is of value in re-educating muscle work and retaining range in such conditions as ankylosing spondylitis.

CHAPTER 10
Springs and Pulleys

M. HOLLIS

Springs are elastic and therefore may have any of the properties of elastic materials. Three of the types of elasticity are used therapeutically, i.e. extensibility, compressibility and torsion.

When springs are extensible they offer resistance to muscle work as they are stretched and as they recoil they offer assistance to movement. During recoil they may be controlled by working muscles in isotonic lengthening.

Compressible springs are used in the form of three springs placed between two halves of hand grip and are used for exercising the gripping muscles of the hand (Figure 96,A). A similar device is a Z-shaped piece of flat spring steel with the flat outer parts of the Z being covered in wood or plastic to form a gripping surface (Figure 96,B). These two types offer resistance by compression.

A third type consists of two handles mounted on straight wires connected together at the end by a coiled spring (Figure 96,C). This type offers resistance by torsion.

These devices are used for increasing the power of the coarse grip. Any type of spring device can be replaced by any compressible material (see section on small apparatus).

Short tension springs of heavy weight resistance have less elasticity and are only suitable for use to give buoyant suspension when a heavy part of the body is to be supported in suspension for a long time.

Long tension springs are the most common type, made in a softer metal and offering weight resistance from 5 kg (approx. 10 lb) to 25 kg (approx. 50 lb) by 5 kg (10 lb) gradations. The weight resistance is marked on a tab attached to the split clips at the ends of the spring and a pull of the marked weight resistance is reached when the cord inside the spring is taut. A pull beyond this length will overstretch the metal and cause deformity by separation of the coils. Such a deformity is also caused by bending springs round plinth ends and by allowing two springs stretched side by side to interlock and remain so.

The method of attaching rings to the split ring end on a spring is shown in Figure 97,A and the method of removal is shown in Figure 97,B.

A carabine is also a very easy method of clipping springs to handles or slings. Some springs are now supplied with a dog clip already attached (Figures 81,A and 81,B).

METHODS OF USE

Rules for the application of forces

The most efficient angle at which a muscle can pull on a bone is one of 90° as then all energy is directed to producing the desired movement. When the angle between the

87

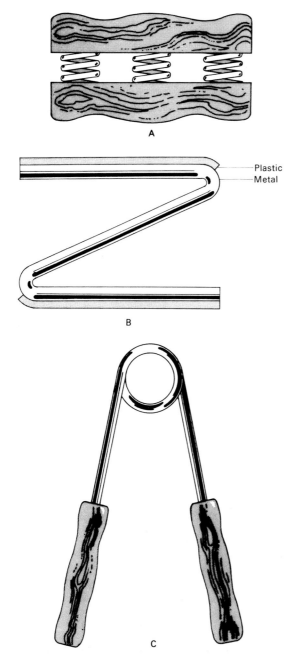

Plastic
Metal

Figure 96 Two types (A and B) of compressible springs; C, A spring offering resistance by torsion.

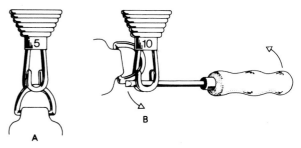

Figure 97 The method of: A, attaching a spring to a split ring; B, detaching a spring from a split ring.

working muscle and the bone is less or greater than 90° some of the energy will be expended in either approximating or separating the joint surfaces. When applying an external force to a moving bone, the same law relating to application of force will operate. Therefore, when force is applied it should be as nearly parallel with the line of movement as is possible and at right angles to the bone. However, as the bones of the body describe an arc of a circle during movement it is only possible to achieve this right angle at one point on the arc; the centre of the arc is usually chosen for the right angle application of the force or the middle range of the contraction of the muscle. In this position the force will be most nearly parallel to the line of motion for the largest part of the arc of motion and the strongest part of the muscle pull. Figures 98,A (90°) and 98,B (165°) show that when force is applied, whether it be a spring or weight and pulley circuit, it is possible to resist a range producing an arc of movement of more than 90° by using two springs each positioned to resist in an arc of movement of 90°. A less effective way of resisting in an arc of movement of 165° would be to position the spring as in Figure

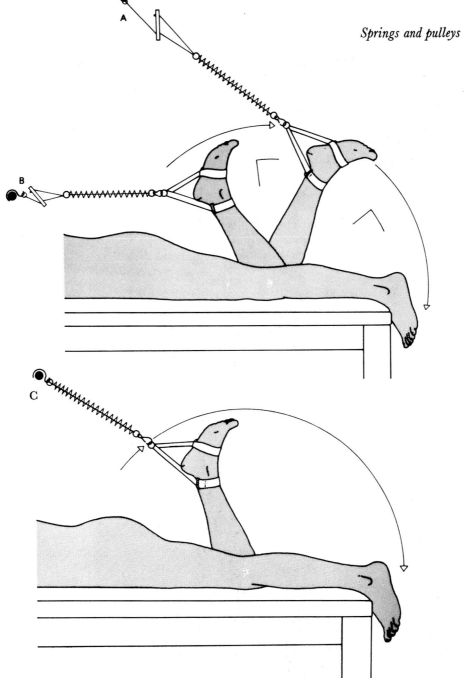

Figure 98 A, The rigging to resist inner range of quadriceps contraction; B, The rigging to resist outer range of quadriceps contraction; C, The rigging to resist the total movement produced by the quadriceps. Maximal only in middle range.

98,C when resistance is maximal in middle range for the quadriceps.

Sometimes it is desired to resist movement of more than one joint, as in extension thrusts of the upper or lower limb, in which case the resistance is applied so as to be parallel to the path of movement of the limb.

It should be noted that when a spring is applied to offer resistance it will *assist* the return movement unless this movement is controlled by the same muscles working in isotonic lengthening. When springs are rigged to offer resistance the following rules should be applied.

1 The patient's starting position should be considered and arranged with sufficient support so that the muscle work occurs where it is required.
2 The movement should be started with the spring slightly stretched and this may also call for modification of the starting position.
3 A suitable weight resistance should be selected relative to:

    a The strength of the muscles.
    b The part being supported and also resisted by the spring, e.g. in Figure 99 the weight of the limb must be supported by the spring when the limb is flexed at the hip and yet it must be possible to achieve full range extension.

4 The correct angle of attachment should be worked out or experimented with to get the resistance in the required range remembering also that the resistance will be greatest when the spring is most fully stretched.
5 To 'lengthen' the distance between the points of attachment a single rope may be used. It should usually be attached to the fixed point and the spring attached either to the sling which is attached to the patient or to the handle which he grips. In this way the patient is more likely to see and hear the spring and sensory stimulation is thereby increased. Exceptions are made when the springs are attached for movements of the head when the noise so near the ears is irritating, or when the spring passes across the naked body and may catch hairs or pinch skin when it recoils.

Spring resistance for the lower limb

Hip abductors These muscles may be worked in Lying and in suspension with the spring attached to the medial side of the foot, or in Yard Grasp Half Standing (Figure 100). A low weight resistance is used as the weight arm is long (try 5–10 kg).

Hip extensors These muscles may be worked in Lying as in Figure 99 when allowance is made for the weight of the leg in selecting the spring (try 15–20 kg) or in Reach Grasp Standing when a much lighter weight resistance is used (try 5–10 kg) (Figure 101).

Hip adductors This group of muscles may commonly need to be re-educated when an above knee amputation has been performed. The patient may be in Lying or, later, in Half Sitting or Standing. The difficulty lies in keeping a sling on the stump. The weight resistance should start low (5 kg) and increase as the patient becomes stronger.

Knee extensors These muscles may be re-

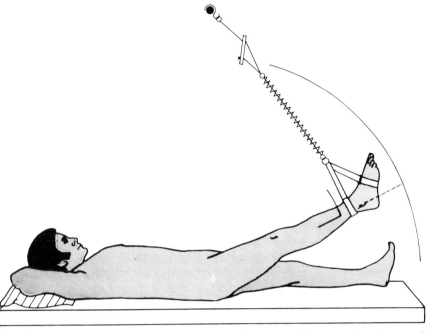

Figure 99　Resistance for the hip extensors. NOTE: The spring must offer enough resistance also to support the limb.

trained in any of the three selected ranges: inner, middle or outer; or simultaneously in all ranges by leaving springs *A* and *B* in Figure 98 in position but reducing the weight resistance as the total resistance offered by both springs will be greater than that by either of them separately.

Knee flexors　The rigging is similar to that for knee extension except that the springs will be resisting in the opposite direction (Figure 102).

Foot plantarflexors　The patient can hold the spring by means of a handle (Figure 103) and so also perform an isometric arm activity. The turns of the three-ring sling must be round the forefoot (try a 10–15 kg spring). Remember here the distance the spring will be pulled out will be small.

Foot dorsiflexors　The turns of the three-ring sling must again be round the forefoot. Try a 5–10 kg spring and prevent cheating by giving the patient a back support. Thus suitable positions are Half Lying or Sitting on a chair with the legs straight and resting on a footstool (Figure 104).

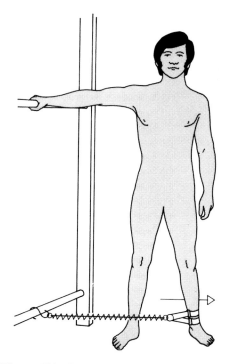

Figure 100   Resistance for the hip abductors.

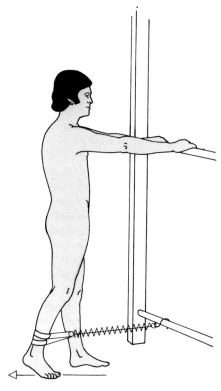

Figure 101   Resistance for the hip extensors.

Foot invertors   These should be rigged as for dorsiflexion but the spring should be attached to the lateral aspect of the foot. Alternatively a three-ring sling may be attached to each foot with a 5 kg spring fixed between them. The patient crosses his knees and he can practise inversion of both feet at once (Figure 105).

Thrusts

If a spring is rigged as in Figure 106 a combined hip and knee extension can be performed and if rigged as shown in Figure 120 hip and knee extension with leg thrusting downwards (lateral pelvic tilting) can be

practised. The same rigging can be used for a hip flexion with knee extension followed by hip extension and slow hip and knee flexion—thus a bicycling movement is done with isotonic shortening and lengthening being performed.

Spring resistance for the upper limb

Shoulder abductors, extensors and flexors.   These muscles can be resisted by putting the patient into Stride Standing and anchoring a sling under his foot on the side of the arm to be

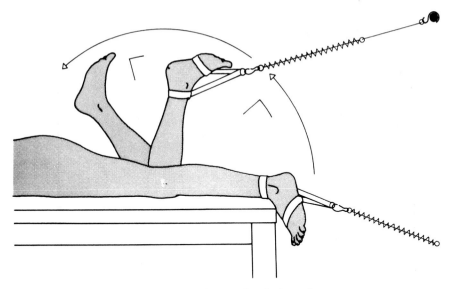

Figure 102   Resistance for the knee flexors.

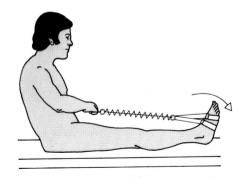

Figure 103   Resistance for the plantarflexors.

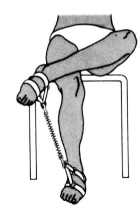

Figure 105   Resistance for the foot invertors.

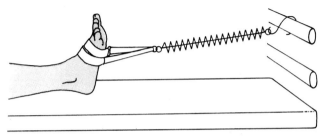

Figure 104   Resistance for the dorsiflexors.

exercised. A 5–10 kg spring is attached to the sling and he holds the other end by means of a handle. Varying the angle at which the arm is raised will allow the same rigging to be used for arm abduction, arm extension, arm flexion and many intermediate movements (Figure 107).

Shoulder rotators   The arm should be supported in a sling attached to a single pulley rope and the patient should hold a handle to which is attached a 5 kg spring. If the other end is attached to the floor below the hand, inner range lateral rotation is resisted and if it is attached to a point above the hand, inner range medial rotation is resisted (Figure 108).

Thrusts for serratus anterior   The patient should be Prone at the edge of the bed and hold a handle attached to a 10 kg spring, the other end of which is attached to a fixed point above his shoulder. He should thrust to the floor protracting his scapula. The same exercise may be performed in Sitting, with the arm supported in slings (Figure 109) if necessary or in Lying with the spring fixed to the floor.

Elbow flexors   The patient is in Toe Support Sitting at the wall bars and holds a spring with a handle. The other end of the spring should be attached in front and to his right for right arm work. He can supinate and flex simultaneously against possibly a 5–10 kg spring.

Elbow extensors   The patient can be Standing or Lying holding a handle with a 10–15 kg spring attached to a point above and behind the head (Figure 110).

Pronators and supinators   Fix two 5 kg springs to a handle, one spring to each of the outer of the three rings on the handle. Stretch both slightly and fix one above and one below the

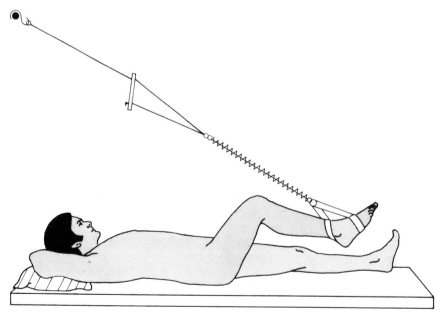

Figure 106   A combined hip and knee extension thrust.

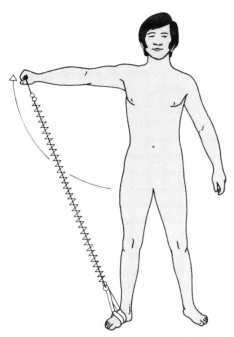

Figure 107 Resistance for the shoulder abductors.

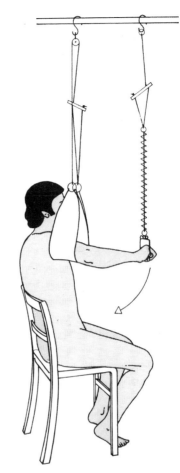

Figure 108 Arm suspension, resistance for the medial rotators of the shoulder.

level of the hand when the elbow is bent. The patient can be Standing or Sitting facing the wall bars. The handle will be held vertical by the tension on the springs and the patient should fix his elbow by tucking it into his waist, grasp the handle and try to **a,** pronate in inner range and **b,** supinate in inner range (Figure 111).

Wrist flexors and extensors Fix a three-ring sling on the palm, attach a 5–10 kg spring. The patient is in Sitting at a table so that his hand is over the far edge of it. The spring may be fixed to the floor level by anchoring it with a sling under the patient's foot. The patient then either supinates the forearm to work the wrist flexors or pronates the forearm to work the

wrist extensors (Figure 112). The three-ring sling should be slipped round on the hand when changing muscle work so that the pull is straight.

Spring resistance for the head and trunk

Head and neck extensors The most usual position for the patient is Lying with a head sling

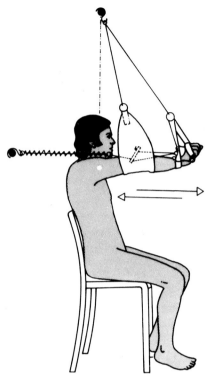

Figure 109 Arm suspension, resistance for serratus anterior. Resisted protraction or resisted forward thrust of whole limb from flexion. In latter case use a lighter spring and omit the rope.

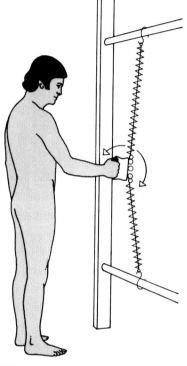

Figure 111 Standing, resistance for the pronators and supinators.

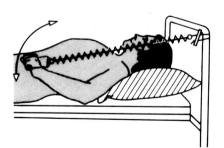

Figure 110 Lying, resistance for the elbow extensors.

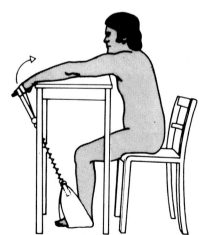

Figure 112 Sitting, resistance for the wrist extensors.

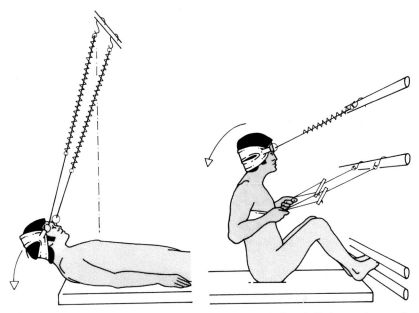

Figure 113 A, Lying, resistance for the head and neck extensors; B, Crook Sitting, resistance for the head, neck and upper back extensors.

under the head, a rope and a 10 kg spring are attached to each side of the sling. The fixed points are head width apart and over the manubriosternal junction to allow for natural flexion. The patient pushes the head backwards when the stool, which initially supports the head, is removed (Figure 113A). Figure 113,B shows an alternative rigging which is harder work and which tends to work the upper trunk extensors as well.

Trunk extensors Figure 114 shows a third method of rigging but the springs must be of heavy resistance (about 20 kg each) and the patient must brace the feet in Crook Sitting with the feet resting on the lowest wall bar. Hip extension will also occur, Figure 115 shows a method of rigging to work the back extensors in inner range.

Trunk flexors The abdominal muscles may be worked as in Figure 116,A by using 10–15 kg springs one to each hand. This has the effect of offering resistance to the abdominal muscles of up to 20–30 kg as the springs are being used in parallel; or with the patient Sitting holding a pole to which are attached two springs (Figure 116,B).

Trunk rotators The springs of similar weight resistance for flexion should be used alternately as in Figure 117 or may be fixed above and behind the patient when he is Sitting on a low-backed chair.

Combined spring resistance

A sequence of bed exercises may be performed

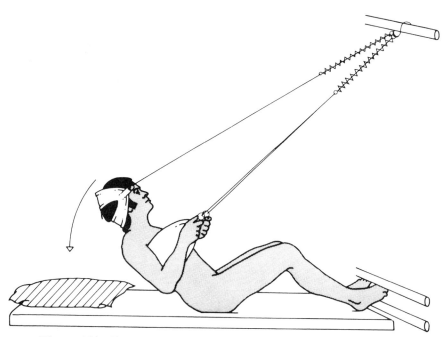

Figure 114 Crook Sitting, resistance for the trunk and head extensors.

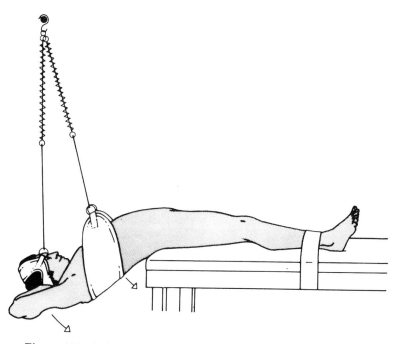

Figure 115 Lying, resistance for the trunk extensors in inner range.

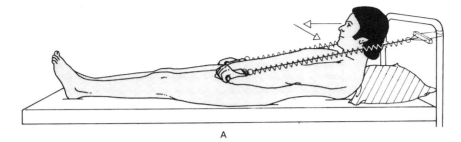

A

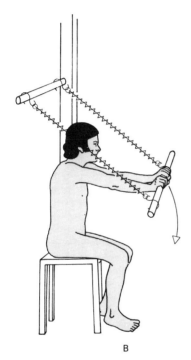

B

Figure 116 A, Lying, resistance for the trunk flexors;
B, Sitting, resistance for the trunk flexors.

in preparation for crutch walking by using the
springs attached to the bed head and

a Working the elbow extensors (Figure 110).
b Continuing to thrust to work the shoulder
depressors.
c Arching the back and working latissimus
dorsi and the back extensors (Figure 118).

d Taking the hands over the thighs, thrusting and raising the head to work the abdominal muscles (Figure 116).
e Thrusting one arm at a time down by the
side and working the trunk side flexors (Figure
119).

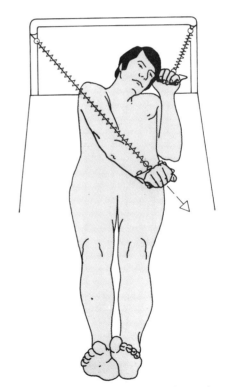

Figure 117 Lying, resisted trunk rotation.

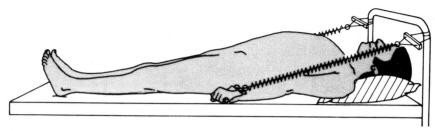

Figure 118 Continued thrust into adduction and extension with back arching works latissimus dorsi and the back extensors.

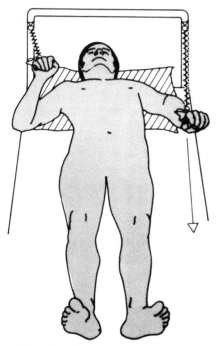

Figure 119 Thrusting with one arm down to the side works the trunk side flexors.

f Thrusting one arm at a time across the trunk and working the trunk rotators (Figure 117).

The above regime is suitable for any long-stay patient who must have lower limb rest or who may have to transfer all activity to the upper limbs and trunk. If eventually the patient will bear weight on one leg then the rigging as in Figure 106 but attached to the bed head will allow

a Leg extension from flexion.
b Bicycling.
c Resisted plantar flexion.
d Thrusting and lateral pelvic tilting.

Three simultaneous limb thrusts as in Figure 120 simulate the 'stance' phase of one leg weight bearing on crutches.

Resisted P.N.F. patterns may be performed using springs provided

a The rigging is suitably arranged.
b The patient is properly instructed and supervised.

PULLEYS

Pulley circuits may be used to change the angle of pull either as auto circuits or as weight and pulley circuits, or to give mechanical advantage, see p. 19.

To change direction of pull

Auto circuit (reciprocal circuit)

The circuit consists of one pulley and a rope

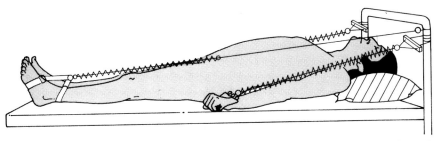

Figure 120 Simultaneous thrust with one leg and both arms as in the 'stance' phase of crutch walking.

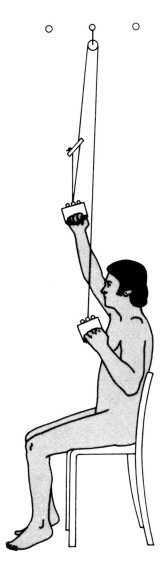

Figure 121 An auto-pulley circuit for reciprocal arm movements.

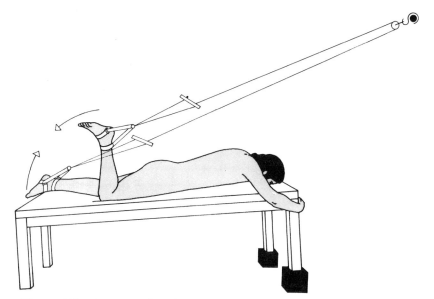

Figure 122   An auto-pulley circuit for reciprocal knee flexion and extension.

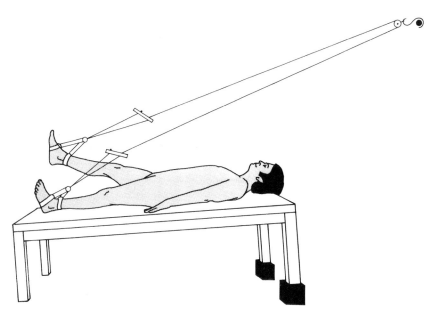

Figure 123   An auto-pulley circuit for reciprocal hip flexion and extension.

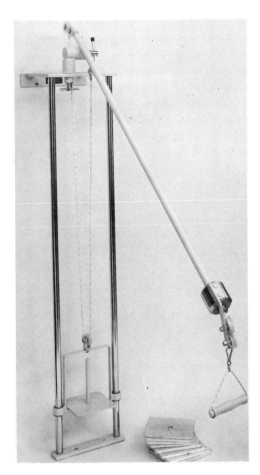

Figure 124 The EMS Rehabilitation Unit. The adjustable arm is mounted on a frame which carries the weight unit. The free end of the arm carries a ball-bearing swivel assembly, through which passes the cord from the arm and weights; and thus to the attachment to the patient.

(Figure 76) with a shortening device and may be used as an auto-pulley circuit for facilitating reciprocal movements of limbs (Figures 121, 122 and 123). In Figures 122 and 123 note the sloping support to allow the body weight to keep the rope taut and prevent cheating.

The method of use of an auto circuit is

a Position the patient to prevent unwanted ('trick') movement.
b The strongest limb or that with the greatest range is put into the position to be achieved by the disabled limb.
c The slings/handles are attached and the rope just tightened.
d The patient is then told to reverse the limb positions slowly initially until he familiarizes himself with the equipment and builds up confidence. Then there are several methods of use.

> **i** Increase the tempo so that the movement is carried past the point of pain by momentum.
> **ii** Tell the patient to make a 'reaching' or overstretch effort at the present limit of his range so that he hurts and helps himself.
> **iii** Teach the patient to use the sound limb to apply the stretch or overpressure, so that if he is caused discomfort it remains within his limit of tolerance.
> **iv** Instruct him to resist each reversal of movement so that he builds up muscle effort and then he can do an extra reach at each end of the cycle of events.

Pulley and weight circuits

More than one pulley in the circuit will allow loading of a movement to occur. Such devices as the Electro Medical Supplies Rehabilitation Unit (Figure 124) allow compact rigging and loading for a variety of movements and muscle work (Figure 125,A,B,C,D). The patient is lifting a known and often visible load and thereby is stimulated to perform better in order to progress to greater loads on succeeding days or weeks.

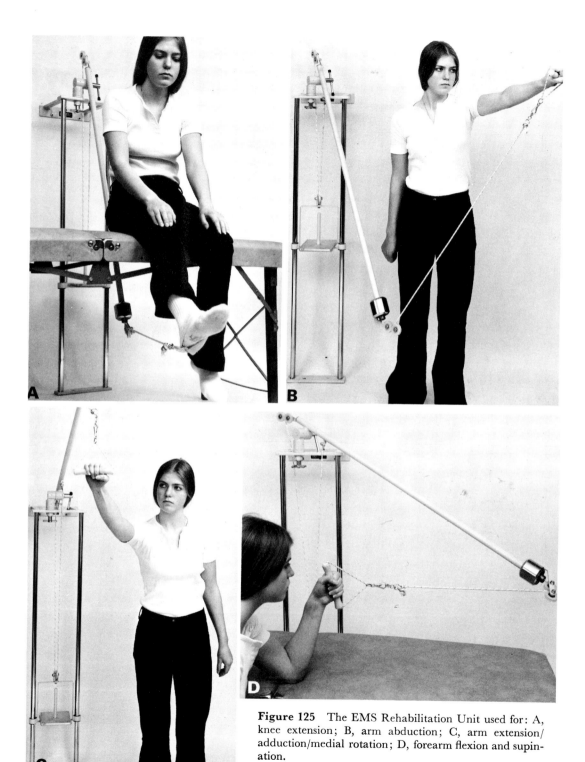

Figure 125 The EMS Rehabilitation Unit used for: A, knee extension; B, arm abduction; C, arm extension/adduction/medial rotation; D, forearm flexion and supination.

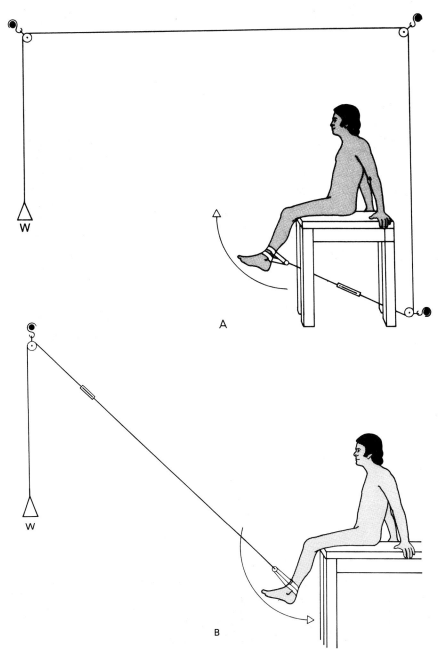

Figure 126 A, A pulley and weight circuit to resist knee extension; B, A pulley and weight circuit to resist knee flexion.

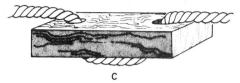

c

Figure 126   C, The 'stop' inserted into pulley and weight circuits.

In the absence of a proprietary device a pulley circuit can be rigged with fixed points as indicated in Figure 126,A,B.

In each of these cases care should be taken to allow the weight to travel up and down without either resting on the ground or hitting the first pulley in the circuit. A 'stop' is also usually introduced in the form of a cleat fitted to the circuit between the patient and the first pulley so that on isotonic lengthening of the muscle, failure of control on the part of the patient does not allow his joint to move through an excessive range (Figure 126,C). This is most important when the patient suffers from both limited range and weak muscles acting over the same joint.

CHAPTER 11

Re-education of Walking

M. HOLLIS

Walking, together with its variants—running, going up and down stairs—is a skilled co-ordinated action which we acquire in infancy and improve with practice. It is an action which involves many joints and muscles, but which is performed by each of us without conscious effort until one of the muscle or joint components involved is disordered. As we walk we move our body components in an orderly manner, adapting to the surface trodden upon and to the space and hazards around us. The whole sensory input is involved and when any part of the sensory system is disordered, gait may also be affected.

Analysis of the disorder and examination of the whole patient may reveal one small cause which, when treated, will resolve the disorder of gait. It is no part of this book to analyse all the gait disorders, but in order to teach the use of walking aids and the return of a patient to the use of normal gait it is necessary to consider all of the muscles and joints which may be involved unless use of a wheelchair is to be a longer term, interim or permanent measure.

The propulsion muscles are the flexors of the toes, the plantarflexors of the ankles, the extensors of the knee and hip.

The 'swing-through' muscles are the extensors of the toes, the dorsiflexors of the ankle, the flexors and extensors of the knee and the flexors of the hip. The abductors and medial and lateral rotators of the hip and side flexors and rotators of the trunk also work in weight transference and pelvic movement. Without adequate pelvic movement in both rotation and hip hitching, correct walking is impossible. The upper trunk and head rotators also work, so that the face and upper trunk maintain a forward facing direction. The range of work of each of these groups will depend upon the length and height of the step.

In consequence of this involvement of many muscles in the act of walking it is necessary to maintain the strength of these muscles and especially those of the weight-bearing limb. In the trunk the additional muscles must also be retrained and/or strengthened and the normal swing of the arms when walking must not be forgotten.

The following regime of exercises should be given to a patient who is in bed and will eventually use crutches or a partial weight-bearing walking aid. All exercises should be resisted by the use of springs or weights when possible and some of those in the sequence may be practised during the course of a ward class or even set to music.

For the arms
gripping
wrist extension
elbow extension
shoulder extension
shoulder medial rotation
shoulder depression

For the trunk
upper trunk—rotation
                    extension
                    flexion
lower trunk—rotation
                    extension
                    flexion
pelvic side flexion or hip hitching.

For the legs
toe and foot flexion and extension
knee flexion and extension
hip flexion and extension
hip abduction and adduction
hip medial and lateral rotation

Some of these exercises may be performed isotonically, others isometrically and some may be performed together. For example, with the patient in slight Crook Lying the therapist may stand at the foot of the bed and, resisting on the soles of the feet, command the patient to perform first a bilateral extension thrust using hip and knee extensors and ankle plantarflexors followed by the reverse movement, with the resistance on the dorsum of the foot. If the resistance is strong enough the patient will slightly extend the lower trunk on the thrust and flex on the pull up. Alternate leg thrusting with a straight hip and knee will cause the patient to perform hip hitching and thus side flex the trunk on the opposite side and use the hip abductor on the thrust side. If the therapist maintains pressure on the soles of the feet or uses a foot board on the bed, or the temperature chart board, then the plantar reflex will be stimulated and the muscles which normally work on the 'stance' phase of walking will all tend to work simultaneously.

Some of the exercises shown in Figures 116,A to 120 are very suitable for the patient to practise alone.

The patients should be encouraged to reach down to the side and across the bed to use their locker and so work the arms and trunk and maintain some balance reactions.

Progression A patient who has spent a long time in the low Half Lying position (three pillows) will take a little time to accommodate to the upright position and should be taught to pull in the abdominal wall or to take several deep breaths to ensure good venous return and an adequate supply of blood to the brain before being sat more upright. Patients who are suspected of poor balance reactions may be given 'Rhythmic Stabilizations' or 'Tapping' (Chapter 25) in Half Lying, Crook Sitting, High Sitting on the side of the bed, feet resting on a stool or preferably in Sitting in a wheelchair in which the patient will feel more secure, to ensure they are ready to start standing practice.

Preparation for walking

The patient should, if possible, be taken to a retraining area fitted with parallel bars and steps. The wheelchair is placed between the parallel bars, the brakes applied, and the patient moved to the front of the chair, the footrests raised and, by pulling with his arms on the parallel bars he is encouraged to stand up bearing weight wherever he is permitted to do so. The therapist should stand at the side and block the standing shoe toe with her instep and the knee of that leg with her knee. She should assist the patient to rise *either* by pressure on the sacrum with one hand and under the axilla of the side more distant from her with the palm (thumb out) of the other hand, *or* by exerting assisting pressure with the axillary grip using the palm only of each hand in the axillae (with the thumb out—one hand across the front to the far axilla, one hand at the back of the near axilla), while blocking the foot and knee from the side. Alternatively the therapist may stand in front of the patient and block the foot with one foot and pull on either the waistband or under the buttocks, thus bringing the patient into standing. The method chosen will depend on the relative heights of patient and therapist, on the stoutness of the patient and the length of the therapist's arms and on the balance ability of the patient.

The patient should now practise balance, and 'Rhythmic Stabilizations' may be practised with pressures on either the shoulders or the pelvis or both. The patient must be encouraged to perform small range flexion and extension of the standing leg and to move the arms in turn forwards and backwards on the bars. If he can bear weight on both legs he should practise transferring his weight first from side to side in Stride Standing and then forwards and backwards in Walk Standing. Pressure from the therapist on the pelvis of the side towards which he is swaying will encourage him to push the pelvis in that direction over the base and so transfer weight to the leg and support of that side. He should be allowed to have several rests as required.

After explanation and perhaps a demonstration he may attempt to progress along the parallel bars using initially a swing-to gait (Figure 134,A) and eventually may be given one or both of his walking aids to use in the parallel bars. He should, if the parallel bars are wide enough, walk first inside them, so that he has something to grasp if he feels unstable. He may use one bar and one walking aid, then both aids, then proceed outside the

bars, but perhaps walk alongside them provided there are no floor obstructions. Eventually he will walk free of the bars but a distance target should be given to him. 'Walk to the door' with the therapist perhaps holding his clothing at the back or putting a steadying hand on his sacrum and one shoulder, until he is more confident and capable of walking with just an escort. The target of distance walked should be constantly revised and the therapist should not hesitate to suggest frequent rests for patients who are afraid, or frail or weak. Equally as the patient performs better and more strongly, not only should the daily distance walked be increased but the rests should be less frequent.

Turning must be taught early unless the bars are of inordinate length and the wheelchair can be taken inside them and, in taking the patient any distance inside or outside the bars it must be remembered that he must traverse a similar distance to return to his wheelchair.

Turning

In the parallel bars The foot is hopped through 45° or less, the now rear arm is moved to the bar the patient is turning to face. A series of hops complete the turn beyond 90° and the arm on the side of the turning direction is moved to behind the patient. Further hops complete the turn.

With walking aids The direction of turn is decided and agreed. The aid on that side is moved backwards and that on the opposite side is moved forwards with a small hop of the appropriate foot as described below. The sequence of moves for a patient weight-bearing on only one leg and turning to the right should be: Right aid back, hop leg to right, left aid forwards, hop leg to right, and repeat until the turn is complete. For a patient weight-bearing on both legs and able to move them separately the sequence for a turn to the right would be: Right aid back, left leg forwards and turned to the right, left aid forwards, right leg back and turned to the right, and repeated to complete the turn.

Some strong patients will complete the process in possibly one or two moves.

Walking up stairs

The patient walks close up to the bottom step, takes his injured limb backwards and, leaning on his walking aids, hops up one step. His walking aids are now brought up on to the same step and the process repeated.

Alternatively he may take both walking aids in one hand and use the banister rail. The procedure is as above, i.e. sound leg first, walking aid last.

Some patients may have to go upstairs backwards on their bottom in which case the hands are put flat on the step above and the trunk raised on to the same step.

Walking down stairs

The patient walks close to the top of the stairs and puts his injured limb in front of himself. He places his walking aids on the step below, lowering by flexing his standing limb. He now hops this limb down to join the walking aids, or he may put both walking aids in one hand and, using the banister rail follow the above sequence of moving his walking aid first and his leg last, or he may sit on the floor and lower his bottom on to the step below his hands.

The disadvantage of climbing up or down

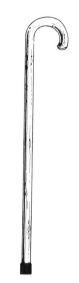

Figure 127   A crook handle wooden stick.

stairs on the bottom is that either two sets of walking aids are needed, one at each end of the flight of stairs, or the aids have to be moved up and downstairs by an assistant or the patient hooking them on to one forearm.

WALKING AIDS

These are appliances which may be a means of transferring weight from the upper limb to the ground or which may be used to assist balance. They fall into the following categories—single point or multipoint, tripod or quadruped (Figures 127–129).

Each point or tip should be rubber or plastic shod with a ferrule of material having a high coefficient of friction and which fits well. Some ferrules are multiringed and depressed to form a vacuum when in contact with the ground, others have multiple small protuberances (Figure 128,A).

All should have a metal washer inside to

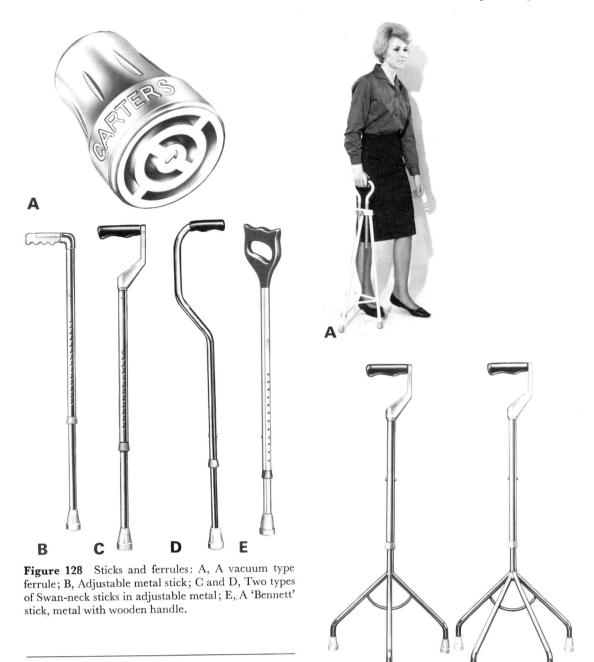

Figure 128 Sticks and ferrules: A, A vacuum type ferrule; B, Adjustable metal stick; C and D, Two types of Swan-neck sticks in adjustable metal; E, A 'Bennett' stick, metal with wooden handle.

Figure 129 A, A tripod correctly used; B, A swan-neck handled tripod; C, A quadripod.

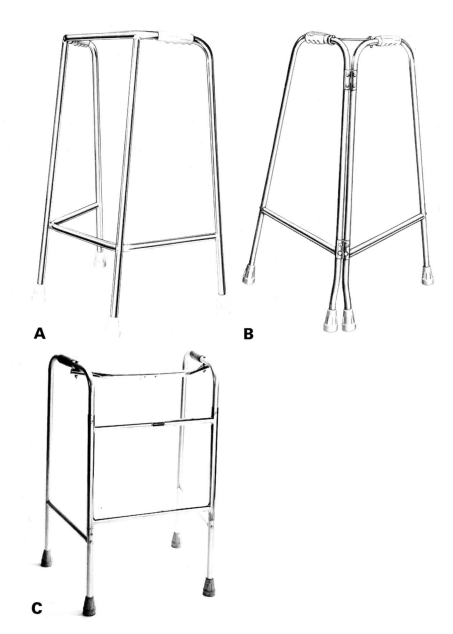

Figure 130   Pick-up aids or frames: A, with three fixed sides; B, with two fixed sides; C, with reciprocal movement of the sides. All three are also made in adjustable heights and different sizes.

prevent the tip of the aid from piercing the ferrule.

Sticks

The upper ends of sticks are of several designs as in Figure 127 and 128,B,C,D,E. The 'crook' top is usually a wooden stick and the flat top and swan-neck top are usually of light metal. Wooden sticks cannot easily have multipoint tips whereas the metal sticks can do so and can also be of adjustable length (Figure 129A,B,C), as can frames (Figure 130,A,B,C).

The correct length of stick allows 15° of flexion at the elbow when the patient is upright, the arm is by the side and the stick is a short distance in front of and to the side of the foot on that side. Measurement is taken with the patient Lying or Standing with the

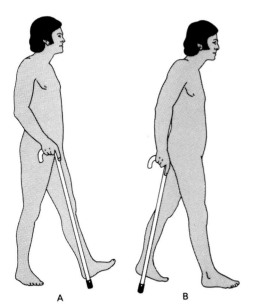

A   B

Figure 131 A and B, The correct positions for a stick in use. The figure shows the correct walking pattern using one stick.

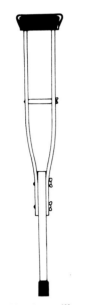

Figure 132   An axillary crutch.

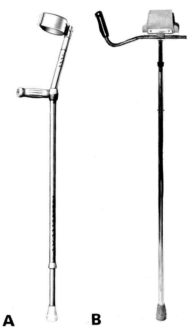

A   **B**

Figure 133 A, An elbow crutch; B, A forearm bearing (gutter) crutch.

arm by the side, from the proximal wrist crease to the shoe heel or the ground 15 cm lateral to the shoe heel. This degree of flexion allows the elbow to straighten when a 'thrust' is made upon the stick as it is used to propel the body forwards. Figure 131,A and B show correct positions for a stick in use.

Crutches

These may also be of wood or metal and should be adjustable both in hand grip to ground length and in axilla to hand grip length.

Axillary crutches   These should be used when weight must be relieved from one leg and can be used to train partial weight bearing before progressing to sticks (Figure 132).

The length is important as the axillary pad must not push up into the axilla, but must be high enough to allow it to be held between the upper arm and the chest wall when weight is put on the crutch. Measurement should be made with the patient's shoes on from the shoe heel to 5 cm below the posterior axillary fold. If the shoes cannot yet be put on, measurement is made from the tip of the medial malleolus to the posterior axillary fold. The position of the hand piece should be adjusted as for a pair of sticks, i.e. to allow 15° of flexion of the elbow when the crutch is held in to the side and is resting 15 cm out from and in front of the shoe toe.

Elbow crutches   These are essentially sticks of adjustable length with a horizontal hand grip and a metal forearm rest which may be in the form of a spring band which is sufficiently elastic to allow the arm to be put through the opening, but tight enough to stay in position on the forearm should the patient release his grip on the hand piece. These crutches are not as stable as axillary crutches, and are more frequently issued for long-term use as, with

practice, it is possible to achieve balance and to let go of a crutch without losing it, in order to perform some manual task, e.g. opening a door, putting shopping in a bag (Figure 133,A).

Forearm bearing (gutter) crutches   These are metal adjustable crutch legs with a gutter splint mounted on the top with, usually, a handle at the front which can be set at an adjustable angle. The forearm is held in the gutter splint by straps of velcro or leather and the hand grips the adjusted handle. These crutches are used when weight cannot be taken through the forearms and hands, e.g. in fractures of these parts or in rheumatoid arthritis of the wrist and hand (Figure 133,B).

Pick-up aids or frames   These are essentially large-based frames having four points and two or three sides. They are used by picking them up, moving them forwards, putting them down, leaning upon them and walking into the frame. They should be adjustable in height (Figure 130,A,B,C). Variations may have:

a   A reciprocal mechanism which allows right hand movement with left leg movement. But this type is often disliked by unsteady patients.
b   Two front legs and two rear casters.
c   Two front legs and two rear wheels with brakes which operate on downward pressure on the wheels.
d   Wheels on all four legs, with or without brakes.
e   'Square' wheels.

The disadvantage of all except the reciprocal frame is that the normal pattern of heterolateral limb movement cannot be used, and they cannot be used up and down staircases.

Crutches may be used to allow mobility when one leg must be non-weight bearing, when both legs may bear weight but cannot propel in normal walking action, or they may be used for partial weight bearing.

The strength and needs of the patient will determine the method of use.

Sticks may be used to relieve a small amount of weight or to help with balance and multipoint pick-up aids are used primarily to help with balance.

PATTERNS OF USE

Crutches

Three-point walking

Swing-to The crutches start in front of the supporting leg. They are lifted and placed further in front, weight is taken on them and the sound leg is bent and swung to just behind the crutches. The disabled leg should be held clear of the ground and in front of the body (Figure 134,A).

Swing-through The above procedure is followed but the sound leg is swung through the crutches and the foot is put down in front of them. This technique is for stronger patients (Figure 134,B).

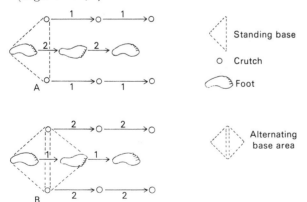

Figure 134 Three-point gait. One leg non-weight bearing. A, The swing-to gait: 1, crutches moved; 2, foot moved. B, The swing-through. The numbers denote the sequence of 'swing-through'.

Both these techniques may be used with any type of crutch.

Four-point walking

Both legs swing-to or swing-through Both legs are swung forwards together and placed either just behind or just in front of the crutches. This technique is more likely to be used by the paraplegic patient and it will depend on his ability and strength whether he will move one crutch at a time, but the legs may be moved together or separately (Figure 135,A,B).

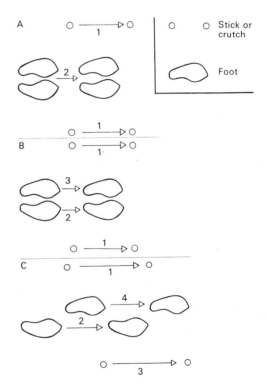

Figure 135 Four-point gaits. Numbers indicate order of swing-through. A, Crutches moved together, both legs moved together. A 'swing-to' pattern; B, Crutches moved together, then each leg in turn. A 'swing-to' pattern; C, Correct walking sequence. One crutch or stick, opposite leg, other crutch or stick, opposite leg.

Three and one pattern   The crutches and partial weight-bearing leg go forward together and the able leg alone while weight is distributed on the other three points which are resting on the ground. This technique is used following non-weight bearing for a limb and when full weight may not yet be taken on an injured limb.

Sticks

Two sticks

a   Both sticks may be taken forward with the injured leg, then the sound leg is brought through. This is a progression on the above type of crutch walking (four-point walking—three and one pattern).

b   The sticks may be used reciprocally in a normal walking pattern. Right stick, left leg, left stick, right leg. Patients sometimes take a little time to achieve this, but its advantage is that the normal walking pattern is used ready for discarding the aids, or is maintained if the aids have to be used for some considerable time (Figure 135,C).

One stick

a   Held on the opposite side from the disablement the walking pattern can be preserved when the only disablement is of one leg. The sequence is—disabled leg and stick, sound leg and free arm swing forward together and in turn (Figure 136,A).

b   Held on the opposite side from the disabled arm and leg. The best pattern is stick and disabled leg, sound leg. The disabled arm may not be able to swing.

Sometimes this proves impossible and a more 'crab–like' gait has to be permitted advancing first the stick, then the sound leg and the disabled leg last. The disabled arm

will trail even more. In these cases a multi-point stick would almost invariably be used (Figure 136,B,C).

c   Occasionally a patient may use one stick in the hand on the same side as the disabled leg. This is commonly done when severely disabling pain is suffered, when the stick and leg are moved forward together.

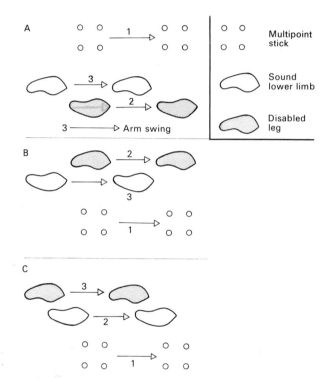

Figure 136   A, A multipoint stick held in the hand opposite to the disabled leg. They move together, then the sound leg and free arm move together; B, A multipoint stick held on the opposite side from the disabled leg and arm. The desirable gait is stick and diabled leg move together then the sound leg. The disabled arm may not be able to swing; C, The stick is held as in B, but the stick and sound leg move together leaving the disabled leg to 'trail' behind. An undesirable gait as the disabled arm will 'trail' even more than in B. The numbers denote the probable sequence of 'swing-through'.

Pick-up aid

The patient puts the aid forwards and walks into it. He should be encouraged to try to take two small even steps—one with each leg in moving into the aid otherwise a more disordered gait may develop.

Wheelchair

Some patients may require exercise while in a wheelchair for temporary disablement, e.g. amputation until weightbearing with confidence and endurance or permanent disablement such as paraplegia. Thus a therapist may be confronted with deciding on the possibility of giving suitable activity to patients of very varying needs who are using a self-propelled wheelchair. After the patient has been introduced to the wheelchair and has learned basic management so that it acts as a substitute for his legs, he may perform other activities from it. The freest exercise and greatest choice of exercise activity can be taken if the chair arms can be removed and the chair back is sufficiently low to allow arm and upper trunk movement, and greater limitations will be imposed if this is not so.

Wheelchair safety The brakes must be efficient, the seat surface must not be too slippy, there should be no adjacent obstructions; the surrounding floor may need to be covered with mats to soften a fall if vigorous exercise is planned. Mechanical factors to be considered not only involve friction (brakes and seat) but the size of the base of the chair related to the patient's height and bulk. A tall, top heavy patient with no leg control and poor balance should not, for example, be encouraged to throw a heavy ball overhead and a long way. This courts loss of equilibrium.

To assess capacity to exercise in a wheelchair ask the following.

> Can the patient grasp and let go?
> Can the patient reach forwards, sideways, upwards and behind (one- or two-handed as appropriate)?
> Can the patient displace and recover the trunk in movements, in trunk rotation, side flexion, flexion and extension?
> Does the patient understand and is he able to perform braking, use of footrests, removal of chair arms, use or removal of special fittings?

From a wheelchair the following may be possible.

> Balance exercises for head, upper trunk, lower trunk.
> Loaded (by weights) exercises for the hands, elbows, shoulders, upper trunk (all movements) leading to ability to lift own body weight in chair.
> Loaded (by pulleys) exercises for the arms and perhaps the knees.
> Loaded (by springs) exercises for the elbow, shoulders, upper trunk, ankles.
> Speed exercises using small apparatus which does not roll away.

When team exercises are used a mixed ability group (some chairbound and some agile) will allow a greater choice of equipment as the agile can act as retrievers.

CHAPTER 12
Examination, Assessment and Recording of Muscle Strength

M. HOLLIS

Muscle malfunction may be easy to identify if disablement is very apparent, on the other hand only complete examination will reveal the exact strength of muscle and its endurance.

Muscle strength is recorded using the Oxford Scale in which:

0 = No contraction is present.
1 = There is a flicker of contraction.
2 = The muscle is capable of performing the full available range of movement with gravity counterbalanced.
3 = The muscle is capable of performing movement against the resistance of gravity into the fullest available range. NOTE: It may not be possible to arrange the patient so that gravity offers resistance throughout the full range. Those muscles which perform over joints having a range much greater than 90° such as the quadriceps or hamstrings will have to be tested through the available gravity-resisted range.
4 = The muscle is capable of performing movement against the resistance of gravity and an added resistance, which should be measured.
5 = The muscle functions normally.

In order to carry out an examination the part should be adequately undressed and compared, if possible, with the other side of the body if it is normal.

Observation will reveal loss of muscle bulk, though this may be irrelevant to loss of power. Passive movement should then be performed to test the passive length of the muscle.

Grades 0, 1 and 2 can be identified by placing the part so that movement can be performed in a gravity neutral situation. The therapist should be able both to see and feel the muscle belly and/or tendon and should not apply manual control to the part moved by the muscle under test, though consideration should be given to placing the muscle in a situation of mechanical and physiological advantage, e.g. use the middle range, ask the muscle to perform its own normal method of working—isotonic shortening or lengthening as the case may be—stretch the muscle slightly first then release the grasp at once. If there is any contraction but little or no movement, then the grade is 1, and if movement through the full available range occurs then the grade is 2.

The position is then changed so that gravity offers resistance to the greatest possible range of movement and again a stretch may be applied before the patient attempts the movement. If the patient can perform a movement through the maximum available range the grade is 3, but care must be taken that in testing for this grade the muscle is isolated and that the patient cannot cheat or perform 'trick' movements.

Grade 4 is tested by using the antigravity

118

position as above and adding a known load in the form of weights (see section on loading). A Grade 4 test may involve testing a 1 Repetition Maximum (1 R.M.). In such a test a muscle is required to lift a maximum load *once* only through most of its range. The 1 R.M. is only used for recording and testing purposes and once performed may exhaust a muscle for a time. A patient should not be required to perform a 1 R.M. more than once weekly.

Normal muscle Grade 5 can perform any of the four roles outlined in group muscle action, i.e. act as agonist, antagonist, synergist and fixator. It can act slowly or quickly and stop as well as start movements. It can work equally well isometrically and isotonically, whether shortening or lengthening, and it has endurance for normal daily activities.

Endurance

This implies the capacity of a muscle to perform normally throughout a day's activities and at the end of the day be no more fatigued than any other muscle in the body. Endurance is tested by subjecting the patients to a full day's activity and observing their state at the end of the day, though in fact endurance may be a subjective assessment made by the therapeutic team consisting of the patient and all those who work with him towards his recovery. It may involve sending him to a rehabilitation and/or training centre where he is subject not only to therapeutic procedures but also to workshop practice both with regard to his working day and the demands of a productive job.

Recording

RECORD OF VOLUNTARY MUSCLE POWER

NAME   DATE OF BIRTH

DIAGNOSIS

RIGHT	Date	UPPER EXTREMITY			Date	LEFT
		Nerve	*Roots*	*Muscle*		
		Accessory	$A_cC_2C_3$	sternomastoid		
			$A_cC_3C_4$	trapezius { upper		
			$A_cC_2C_3C_4$	middle		
			$A_cC_2C_3C_4$	lower		
		Brachial plexus	$C_3C_4C_5$	levator scapulae		
			C_4C_5	rhomboids		
			$C_5C_6C_7$	serratus anterior		
			$C_5C_6C_7C_8T_1$	pectoralis major		
			$C_4C_5C_6$	supraspinatus		
			C_5C_6	intraspinatus		
			$C_6C_7C_8$	latissimus dorsi		
			C_6C_7	teres major		

RIGHT	Date	UPPER EXTREMITY			Date	LEFT
		Nerve	*Roots*	*Muscle*		
		Axillary	C_5C_6	teres minor		
			C_5C_6	deltoid { anterior		
			C_5C_6	middle		
			C_5C_6	posterior		
		Musculus cutaneus	C_5C_6	biceps brachii		
			C_5C_6	brachialis		
		Radial	$C_6C_7C_8$	triceps { long hd.		
			$C_6C_7C_8$	lateral hd.		
			$C_6C_7C_8$	medial hd.		
			$C_5C_6C_7$	brachioradialis		
			C_6C_7	ext. carpi rad. long.		
			C_7C_8	ext. carpi rad. brev.		
			C_5C_6	supinator		
			C_7C_8	extensor digitorum		
			C_7C_8	ext. digiti minimi		
			C_7C_8	ext. carpi ulnaris		
			C_7C_8	abd. pollicis longus		
			C_7C_8	ext. pollicis longus		
			C_7C_8	ext. pollicis brevis		
			C_7C_8	ext. indicis		
		Median	C_6C_7	pronator teres		
			C_6C_7	flex. carpi radialis		
			C_7C_8	palmaris longus		
			$C_7C_8T_1$	flex. dig. superficialis		
			C_8T_1	flex. dig. prof. 1 & 2		
			C_8T_1	flex. pollicis longus		
			C_8T_1	abd. pollicis brevis		
			C_8T_1	opponens pollicis		
			C_8T_1	flex. pollicis brevis		
			C_8T_1	lumbrical 1		
			C_8T_1	2		

RIGHT	Date	UPPER EXTREMITY			Date	LEFT
		Nerve	*Roots*	*Muscle*		
		Ulnar	C_7C_8	flex. carpi ulnaris		
			C_8T_1	flex. dig. prof. 3 & 4		
			C_8T_1	abd. dig. minimi		
			C_8T_1	opp. dig. minimi		
			C_8T_1	flex. dig. min. brev.		
			C_8T_1	lumbrical 3		
			C_8T_1	4		
			C_8T_1	interossei palmar 1		
			C_8T_1	2		
			C_8T_1	3		
			C_8T_1	4		
			C_8T_1	dorsal 1		
			C_8T_1	2		
			C_8T_1	3		
			C_8T_1	4		
			C_8T_1	add. pollicis		

Notes:

NAME   DATE OF BIRTH

DIAGNOSIS

RIGHT	Date	LOWER EXTREMITY			Date	LEFT
		Nerve	*Roots*	*Muscle*		
		Femoral	$L_1L_2L_3$	ilio-psoas		
			L_2L_3	sartorius		
			$L_2L_3L_4$	quadriceps { rect. fem.		
			$L_2L_3L_4$	vast. lat.		
			$L_2L_3L_4$	vast. med.		
			$L_2L_3L_4$	vast. inter.		
		Obturatori	$L_2L_3L_4$	add. longus		
			$L_2L_3L_4$	add. magnus		
			L_2L_3	gracilis		
		Inf. glut.	$L_5S_1S_2$	gluteus maximus		

RIGHT	Date	LOWER EXTREMITY			Date	LEFT
		Nerve	*Roots*	*Muscle*		
		Sup. gluteal	$L_4L_5S_1$	gluteus medius		
			$L_4L_5S_1$	gluteus minimus		
			L_4L_5	tensor fasciae latae		
				lateral rotator group		
		Sciatic	$L_5S_1S_2$	semimembranosus		
			$L_5S_1S_2$	semitendinosus		
			$L_5S_1S_2$	biceps femoris		
		Tibial	S_1S_2	gastrocnemius		
			S_1S_2	soleus		
			L_4L_5	tibialis posterior		
			S_2S_3	flex. dig. longus		
			S_2S_3	flex. hall. longus		
		Deep peroneal	L_4L_5	tibialis anterior		
			L_5S_1	ext. dig. longus		
			L_5S_1	ext. hallucis		
			L_5S_1	ext. dig. brevis		
		Sup. peroneal	$L_5S_1S_2$	peroneus longus		
			$L_5S_1S_2$	peroneus brevis		
		Plantar	S_2S_3	abductor hallucis		
			S_2S_3	lumbricals		
			S_2S_3	interossei		

RIGHT	Date	TRUNK			Date	LEFT
		Nerve	*Roots*	*Muscle*		
		Intercostal	T_{1-6}	intercostals upper		
		Intercostal	T_{7-12}	intercostals lower		
		V.R.	T_{6-12}	rectus abdominis		
		V.R.	T_{6-12}	ext. abd. oblique		
		V.R.	$T_{7-12}L_1$	int. abd. oblique		
		D.R.	$C_{3-8}T_{1-12}L_{1-5}$	erector spinae		
		Lumbar plexus	$T_{12}L_1L_2L_3$	quadratus lumborum		
		D.R.	$C_{4-8}T_{1-12}L_{1-5}$	intrinsic back muscles		

Notes:

Re-education of muscle

When a muscle which has apparently lost all power is to be re-educated it is necessary to give it both physiological and mechanical advantage so that if it is possible for the muscle to contract it will be able to do so.

Mechanical advantage may be offered by positioning the patient so that either gravity offers assistance to the movement which the muscle normally performs or preferably so that the part is in a position in which gravity is *neutral* and offers neither resistance nor assistance to the movement to be performed.

The patient should have a demonstration of the movement which is to be performed and should watch intently whilst this is being done. Clearly audible commands and instructions should be given before and during the training regime.

The movement should be done in middle range if this is the point at which the muscle will act at right angles to its bony attachment. A choice will have to be made between either an isotonic shortening or an isotonic lengthening as the first attempt at muscle action and it is more usual to choose the *normal* activity of the muscle; if normal activity is an isometric contraction then this is used with the therapist's hand offering resistance in the normal position in the range in which the muscle normally contracts isometrically.

The therapist's hands should be placed so that one can control the proximal part, i.e. the origin of the muscle and the joints proximal to this part and so that the same hand can palpate the muscle belly.

The more distal hand will have to carry out several functions. In the first place it must offer resistance, especially so if a gravity-assisted movement is being used. The distance along the limb at which this hand is placed will control the length of the weight arm. Secondly, it may possibly have to initiate the movement, as it may be feasible for a muscle to continue a movement once inertia has been overcome; and thirdly this hand will have to introduce some of the all-important physiological factors which facilitate the muscle's contraction. In other words—pressure on the 'leading' surface and stretch to the muscle to be worked will be applied by the distal hand.

With the patient concentrating mentally and having a mental picture of the movement to be performed, looking to see what is happening, listening to the therapist's clear commands and the muscle being stretched rapidly immediately prior to the command to work, then there will be physiological summation of stimuli at the anterior horn cells supplying that particular muscle, more especially so if the muscle can contract and resistance can continue to be offered throughout the active movement.

Timing is very important at this point in the proceedings as the therapist must apply the stretch and immediately move the part so that the muscle can operate at a maximally satisfactory angle of pull and she must also immediately, if necessary, change the pressure on the part so that she resists, not assists, the movement. Practice will make the therapist more skilled in this particular technique.

Progression

Progress can be made in one of several ways based on the above points.

a The range through which the muscle works may be increased gradually.
b The amount of resistance offered by the therapist may be increased gradually.
c The length of the weight arm may be increased gradually.
d The muscle may be required to initiate

the movement as well as to continue to perform it.

e The muscle may be required to work both in isotonic shortening and in isotonic lengthening in succession. This may be termed two-way innervation or continuous demand. The muscle is thus increasing its endurance as it is now working for twice the length of time of a single one-way contraction.

f The muscle may be required to work isometrically at different points in the range. When the muscle can perform an isometric contraction as a true 'hold' it can be required to act as part of a team. That is it can undertake each of the activities of group muscle action. By this time it would be anticipated that a muscle would be capable of carrying out a contraction at about Grade 2 on the Oxford Scale.

There is no reason whatsoever why, during the stage of recovery prior to this point being reached, the muscle should not be stimulated by being included in group activity or mass movement patterns as described in Chapters 22 to 24. When this is done the mass movement pattern is more usually done by the stronger proximal muscles which are then required to 'hold' (isometric muscle work) at the strongest point in the mass movement whilst the therapist 'plays' on the paralysed or weak muscle—stretching it, concentrating the patient's attention on it and attempting to make it participate in the mass activity. If the therapist succeeds in persuading the muscle to work then the remainder of the mass movement pattern is continued, with the muscle included in the activity but the quantity of resistance offered to the weak muscle will be less than that offered to the stronger muscles in the pattern of mass movement.

When a muscle is learning to work as both

an agonist and as an antagonist then the technique known as 'Slow Reversals' is used. The muscle first works as an agonist and then, without pause, the movement is reversed so that the opposite muscles work and the former working muscle now relaxes reciprocally.

The muscle may do this in single joint movement such as flexion and extension of the elbow or in a mass or group movement pattern such as taking the arm from the extension/abduction/medial rotation position to the flexion/adduction/lateral rotation position with the associated movements of the elbow, radioulnar, wrist, finger and thumb joints (associated flexion of elbow, supination and flexion of wrist and fingers). In this example biceps brachii can thus be re-educated in its flexion of elbow/supinator role and also as a flexor of the shoulder via its short head; or the extension/adduction/medial rotation pattern with its associated movements may be used for opponens pollicis to be re-educated in its 'grasp' function.

A muscle needs to be re-educated at frequent intervals during the day so that short bursts of treatment are given rather than one long treatment in which the muscles and the patient become over fatigued. A well-planned programme of re-education would start with the strongest group of muscles to be retrained, continuing with the weaker groups and move from one to another part of the body so that each affected part is treated in turn, rests while another part works and then there is a return to work the strongest part again.

In addition to re-education of single actions, muscles must be re-educated to work in patterns, so that perhaps the first treatment may be of single actions, the second treatment of group or mass patterns (see Chapters 22 to 24), the third treatment may be in a change of medium, e.g. in the hydrotherapy pool with single and oblique patterns combined, whilst the fourth treatment could be a functional activity in which the weak muscle has to undertake perhaps objective work repetitively in order to increase endurance.

A programme such as this will not be possible for a very weak muscle below Grade 2 on the Oxford Scale, but once a muscle has achieved Grade 2 then effort and endurance can rapidly be progressed through a programme as outlined above. In addition to the manual loading which the therapist will apply and constantly adjust, a regime of mechanical loading can be started.

Thus, first gravity is the resistance, then the weight arm is lengthened, then as weights are added to the part the weight arm may be first shortened and again lengthened.

Once a weight can be applied to a part it is important to use a weight which is known and recordable and a training regime for which the patient is partly responsible. The 10 Repetition Maximum (10 R.M.) is found for each muscle or muscle group. It can be estimated in several ways.

a   Use is made of a spring balance which is attached so that it is at right angles to the middle of the arc of movement produced by the muscle. An effort is made by the patient to stretch the spring balance and a reading is taken. Three efforts are usually made and the average result taken as the 10 R.M.
b   The 10 R.M. may be known, as the training regime may have started with, for example, a $\frac{1}{2}$ kg weight and been increased daily.
c   The therapist may place her hand on the part and ask the patient to make an effort against her resistance. If she then immediately takes sandbags in her hand until she feels the same 'load', then this weight can be used as the 10 R.M.

If the patient can make ten efforts with that weight and the muscle just quivers with fatigue on the tenth attempt then the therapist has made a correct estimate. If the muscle quivers after less than ten attempts the load is too heavy and if it does not quiver on the tenth attempt then the load is too light. After a rest the load should be adjusted and a further attempt should be made.

Once the 10 R.M. is known there are three training regimes which may be used.

1   De Lorme and Watkins
   10 lifts of half 10 R.M.
   10 lifts of three-quarters 10 R.M.
   10 lifts of 10 R.M.
   30 lifts four times weekly. Retest the 10 R.M. once weekly.
2   Macqueen
   10 lifts of 10 R.M. repeated four times—total of 40 lifts three times weekly. The 10 R.M. is progressed every 1–2 weeks.
3   Zinovieff or Oxford
   10 lifts of 10 R.M.
   10 lifts of 10 R.M.—$\frac{1}{2}$ kg.
   10 lifts of 10 R.M.—1 kg.
   10 lifts of 10 R.M.—$1\frac{1}{2}$ kg.
   10 lifts of 10 R.M.—2 kg.
   10 lifts of 10 R.M.—$2\frac{1}{2}$ kg.
   10 lifts of 10 R.M.—3 kg.
   10 lifts of 10 R.M.—$3\frac{1}{2}$ kg.
   10 lifts of 10 R.M.—4 kg.
   10 lifts of 10 R.M.—$4\frac{1}{2}$ kg.
   100 lifts fives times weekly. The 10 R.M. may be progressed daily, but the 1 R.M. is usually tested and recorded less frequently. It is purely a measure of progress. If the 10 R.M. is less than 5 kg. then reductions are made by making use of $\frac{1}{4}$ kg and $\frac{1}{2}$ kg units. Endurance is built up by the use of lesser resistances than the 10 R.M. and a higher repetition regime.

Although these regimes are most commonly used for building up large groups such as the extensors of the knee using a weight directly applied, there is no reason whatever why the repetition maxima type of programme should not be used using a pulley and weight circuit or using a spring as the resistance.

In addition muscle re-education in circuit training must be included as part of the daily regime. Circuit training will have the advantage that a specially devised system of exercises for that particular patient with those especially weak muscles, will make those muscles work in a functional way. It will load the muscle in different ways, will give the patient a regime he can practise alone and in which he can aim at a weekly improvement in performance.

Circuit training

This is a means whereby a patient is given a series of exercises to be performed regularly, e.g. weekly in a gymnasium or several times a week in a gymnasium, or up to three times a day unsupervised.

The object of using a circuit is to improve cardiovascular performance and muscular endurance. Regular testing and recording is essential. This involves both patient and therapist in some paper work especially in setting up the initial circuit.

A circuit usually consists of between six and eight exercises and may vary from simple, free exercises to those involving the use of as many pieces of apparatus as there are exercises in the circuit.

Each patient must learn to perform each exercise adequately before he is allowed to use it in his circuit and to this end uncomplicated exercises should be given. Circuits are not measures of skill and it is better to

have good performance of an easier exercise than poor and reducing performance of a more complex exercise.

Circuits may be arranged either for activity of the whole body to build up general fitness and endurance or may be aimed at a more specific objective, e.g. strengthening one group of muscles by making those muscles work in several different ways: slowly and with control, fast, heavily loaded, associated with more distal muscles, associated with more proximal muscles and in a whole-body activity. It is usual to keep the number of repetitions of each exercise at a figure between five and thirty.

When devising circuits with a high apparatus content the timing must be carefully organized to prevent bunching and queuing. Apparatus circuits or very difficult circuits may be graded, usually into three divisions when the number of repetitions of each exercise controls the degree of difficulty.

If a fixed equipment circuit is to be set up it is possible to devise large cards to be placed in clear view beside the apparatus. These carry the following information.

The *name* of the exercise.
The *number* of the exercise in the circuit.
An *outline drawing* of the exercise.
The *number of repetitions* to be done by each *grade* of participant (usually in three different colours—one for each grade).
The *name* and *place* of the *next* exercise.

Each participant needs a card indicating his grade (by colour), the exercise numbers and a date of each attendance. He inserts the number of performances of each exercise on that day and when he reaches an agreed level he is retested and/or regraded to a higher grade.

Circuits can be of three main types:

Fixed time circuits in which a certain number of exercises, usually six, are performed, each one of them for a limited time, usually 1 minute with a 1 minute rest between each exercise. The number of times the patient performs each exercise is counted and recorded when the circuit is first given and then re-counted weekly. The daily performance should consist of the circuit of exercises performed without conscious rest and repeated three times in succession. The number of repetitions of each exercise need not be the test rate, but should be an agreed lesser rate initially and the patient should attempt to gain a higher repetition rate in the third run through the circuit and try gradually to increase the number of repetitions of each run through the circuit. If improvement has occurred the number of times each exercise is performed per minute will have increased. This type of circuit increases endurance.

Fixed repetition circuits, in which, usually, six exercises are each performed for 1 minute on the test day with a 1 minute rest between. The number of times each exercise is done is recorded and the patient then repeats the regime doing each exercise the test number of times without conscious rest and the circuit three times. On retesting after 7 days it may be found that the total performance time for the circuit has dropped to less than 6 minutes. This type of circuit tends to increase strength slightly more than endurance.

Progression of a fixed time circuit is made by allowing the patient to achieve the maximum number of repetitions which will be indicated by the same result on two successive weeks and then changing that exercise for a more difficult one. A fixed repetition circuit is progressed by increasing the number of repetitions on the test day until a minute has elapsed and this is the new daily target for each exercise. Again, when the patient cannot increase the number of repetitions of any exercise in a minute the limit has been reached, and that exercise should be made more difficult.

Beginners circuits with progressions This type of circuit is more useful for groups of very mixed ability patients when each person in the group must do the same exercises. The therapist teaches the exercises to everyone, in circuit order, and fixes the circuit time using knowledge gained from the teaching; this time should be approximately that in which a good performer may complete three laps of the circuit at half the maximum repetitions as determined in a fixed repetition circuit. Lower repetitions are then given to the less able performers. The repetition numbers are put on cards for each exercise in the circuit and the cards can be put up in the gymnasium or handed to each patient. Each patient performs his own number of repetitions of the exercises in the circuit, does each circuit three times, checks and records his performance time. As each patient reduces his performance time to less than that estimated for his grade (e.g. Beginner, Middle and Fit) he should move up a grade. The Fit patient increases his repetitions to three-quarters and then to the maximum number of repetitions aiming at performing them in the original estimate of circuit time.

Patients should be told exactly when to do the circuits and to eliminate doubt should be given a card with the regime written down. It is advisable to check that he has sight of a suitable clock for the fixed time and beginners' regimes, and it sometimes helps if patients are paired and act as counters or timekeepers for each other. They should be

Sample table of exercises for Fixed Time Circuit, e.g. for knee injuries

Test time of 11 minutes; 6 exercises of 1 minute each and 5 rests of 1 minute each

Exs. No.	Exercise name	Test No. of repetitions 20th Oct.	Rep. 1	Rep. 2	Rep. 3	Test No. of repetitions 27th Oct.
1	Sit down and stand up	30	20	25	30	
2	Run on the spot w. High Kn. raise	40	20	30	40	
3	Step St. to ½ High St. w. ¼ turn round stool	24	15	18	24	
4	Skipping	24	16	20	24	
5	High Jump to touch target	8	6	7	8	
6	Run as far as possible in 1 minute	200 yds	200 yds	200 yds	200 yds	
		Recorded by a counter	Recorded by patient on day of exercise			Recorded by a counter

Sample table of exercises for fixed apparatus circuit

(This is also a fixed repetition circuit)

Exs. No.	Exercise Name	Repetition No. for		
		Beginner	Middle	Fit
1	Std. St. A. Bd. and Str. u. w. wt.	10	20	30
2	½ St. Hop in and out of hoop	6	15	25
3	Rch. Gsp. Ly. (under beam). Pull ups	6	12	20
4	Wk. St. Bd. to pick up quoit and post in wall bar	8	16	30
5	Toe. Supp. Ly. Sitt. ups.	6	15	25
6	Run up and down inclined form to touch targets u. an d.	8	16	25

Fixed Time Circuit: Patient's Record

Exs. No.	Day 1			Day 3			Day 5			Day 1			Day 3			Day 5		
	X	X	X	X	X	X	X	X	X	X	X	X	X	X	X	X	X	X
1																		
2																		
3																		
4																		
5																		
6																		

advised that it is important that they complete each circuit without resting and that they record accurately for themselves.

The value of circuits lies not only in the increase of the patient's endurance and strength but in their flexibility in use and the transfer of the responsibility for his performance entirely to the patient. A young fit man with a knee injury can do a circuit alongside a chronic bronchitic as each of them is performing to his own limit but within the same rules.

Muscle loading

A muscle will work maximally if it is maximally loaded, i.e.

$$\text{work} = \text{load}$$

Thus when work is demanded of a muscle it should be given maximum resistance in order to produce fatigue. Fatigue is indicated by:

a A slower response to command.
b A slower or lesser range of performance.
c Quivering of the muscle belly.
d No action—this is extreme fatigue and rarely occurs in the incapacitated except when a paralysed muscle recovers and 'flickers' for the first time since onset of paralysis.

A muscle may be loaded in many ways, and the therapist will have to decide at which point to build up strength by maximal loading associated with low repetitions or endurance by a lesser loading associated with frequent repetitions.

There are three regimes which may be used for self practice (see p. 120). However, these require first an estimation of the 10 R.M. and then its weekly reestablishment. The advantage of these regimes is that the performance of each is patient triggered and controlled, once the patient has been taught what to do and he can use one of these regimes as part of a programme of treatment. One disadvantage is that maximal effort can be avoided by poor endeavour. Another is that patients often progress much faster than the orthodoxy of the regimes allows for. When this happens the therapist should use the principles of establishing the load and train the patient to use a regime compatible with his needs and the aims of his treatment.

Manual loading

The greatest advantage of manual loading of any muscle work, whether a single muscle or a group or a whole pattern of action, is that the therapist can use her own hands both to stimulate effort and to palpate and be continually aware of the patient's response; thus a variable resistance can be offered in accordance with the varying strength of the muscle/s as it works in its various ranges and with differing capacities according to its quality of strength and degree of fatigue.

Self loading

This is also called auto loading and is brought about when a patient offers self-resistance to his own muscle actions. These may be in three ways,

a By offering resistance to the movement of one part of the body by resisting directly with another part, e.g. the right arm resisting the upward movement of the left arm, or the right leg crossed at the ankle over the left offering resistance to knee extension. In both the examples quoted the movement is also occurring against the resistance of gravity. Similarly auto-resisted pulley circuits may be used (see Chapter 10).
b Movement of the body weight itself may be called auto loading as in Standing slowly bending and straightening the hips and knees.
c By performing a movement in such a

manner that it is weighted by the intensity of the muscle action. Slow dramatic movements will self load a muscle action.

Variable loading

By using a spring as a resistance the work performed by the muscle can be varied as the spring will offer maximal resistance only when it is maximally stretched. The muscle may not put the same effort into each contraction. Moreover, the recoil of the spring may either return the part to a resting position with no effort from the muscle or may be controlled by the muscle thus performing an isotonic lengthening. In other words the more control the patient exerts on the spring the greater the muscle effort and the longer it will be performed as the muscle must first shorten isotonically and then lengthen isotonically.

Weight loading

This is a type of loading which may be applied

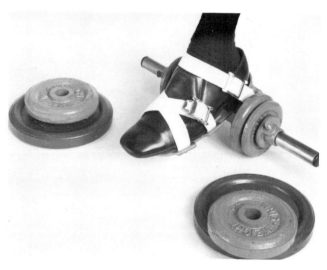

Figure 137   The Variweight boot.

directly to a part by placing a weight in a suitable position using either a special device such as the Variweight or de Lorme type boot (Figure 137) or a bar, a barbell, a sandbag or a bag of shot. Alternatively a pulley and weight circuit may be used as in Figures 124 to 126 or the type like the apparatus (Figures 126,A,B) in which the weight can be placed so that it can be seen to move whenever the patient makes an effort.

The advantage of any of these types of loading is that the patient is moving a known weight with every endeavour. The disadvantages are that secure anchorage is sometimes difficult to achieve and the patient may not make a maximal effort at each attempt.

Any one of the three regimes outlined on page 120 may be used in this type of loading.

Techniques

Using the de Lorme type or Variweight boot   This consists of a metal foot plate and straps weighing 500 g. A bar of varying weight may be supplied and it is essential to know the weight of the bar in calculating the load. The boot may be used for loading the quadriceps or hamstrings when the bar is placed in the rear slots on the foot plate and anchored by *both* of the securing screws. For loading dorsi- or plantarflexion of the foot, the bar is placed in the front slot on the foot plate and anchored by *one* screw.

The order of events in applying the boot is:

a   Position the patient correctly supporting the distal part initially.
b   Apply the unloaded boot and secure it to the patient's shoe.
c   Position and fix the bar.
d   Load the weights equally on each side of the bar.

e   Secure them with the end stops which must be screwed into position so that the weights cannot move.
f   Remove the limb support if necessary and immediately require performance of the exercise.

The quadriceps are exercised with the

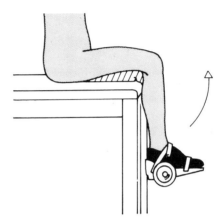

Figure 138   High Sitting, quadriceps exercise using the Variweight boot.

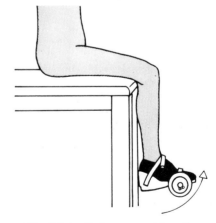

Figure 139   High Sitting, exercising the anterior tibial muscles. Note the bar is to the front of the boot.

patient in High Sitting on a backward-sloping surface preferably padded under the knee (Figure 138) so that the body acts as a counter-weight and the patient does not slip forward.

The anterior tibials are exercised in the same position but a back slope is not so necessary (Figure 139). In both the above cases the limb should be supported on a stool until the boot and weights are fixed and the stool should be re-inserted under the boot at the end of the performance.

The hamstrings are exercised with the patient in Prone Lying but the range of movement allowed at the knee should be just less than 90° (Figure 140) and it may be necessary to change the length of the bar at each side of the boot to take into account variations in strength between the medial and lateral hamstrings.

The plantarflexors are also exercised in the Prone Lying position. In both the above cases the foot should rest over the end of the support (Figure 141).

In using a de Lorme boot for treatment of the thigh muscles the foot is the area to be loaded and the anterior tibials and calf muscles must have adequate power to tolerate

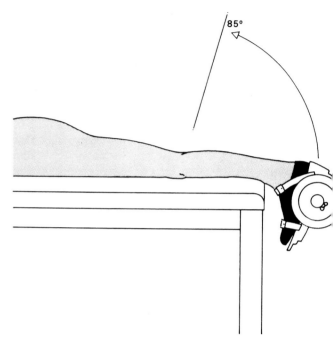

Figure 140   Prone Lying, hamstring exercise using the Variweight boot.

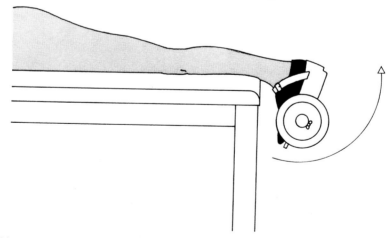

Figure 141   Prone Lying, exercising the calf muscles. Note the bar is to the front of the boot.

the load. This equally applies if a sandbag is placed on this region. Direct loading of the hamstrings or quadriceps only can be obtained by using a weight and pulley circuit and fixing the sling to the lower leg above the ankle joint (Figure 126,A,B).

Using weights of canvas and sand or shot The canvas should be strong and of closely woven mesh and should be double stitched at the edges to keep the fine contents in place. The total weight of canvas and contents should be marked on each container—usually 500 g, 1 kg, 1·5 kg, 2 kg, 3 kg, 5 kg. Two styles are made.

a A bag (Figure 142,A) having a flat area at one end in which a metal eyelet hole is inserted allowing the weight to be suspended.
b A saddle in which a long strip of canvas has weights in pockets at each end. The centre (unloaded) area rests on the part to be loaded. Half the total contents should be inserted in each end of the saddle (Figure 142,B). The advantage of this type is that it can be laid

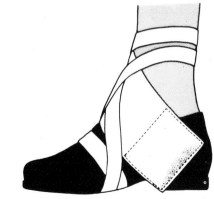

Figure 143   A, A saddle weight held on the foot by the use of a band repeatedly crossed.

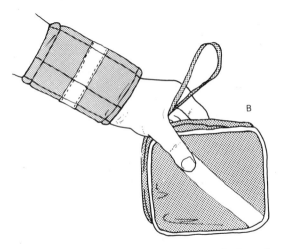

Figure 143   B. A Portabell weight attached to the wrist. The carrying case is also shown.

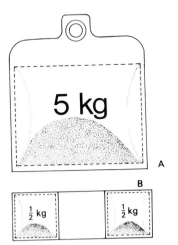

Figure 142   A, A canvas bag weight; B, A canvas saddle weight.

across the area to be loaded or the unloaded centre portion may be grasped.

Fixing weights such as sandbags to the lower limb can be done by using a band. The band is placed round the back of the ankle. The weights are placed on the front of the ankle and held in position by crossing the hand in front of them. By crossing the band under the foot and continuing to cross the band around the foot the full length of the band is used up and the weights will be firmly secured (Figure 143,A).

Using weighted bands 'Portabell' weights are weighted bands made of artificial fibre fastened with velcro. The bands have pockets in which lead shot is placed and they are made in two sizes and weights, 1¾ lb and 2½ lb. They are supplied in pairs in a carrying case (Figure 143,B).

The bands are placed round the limb to be exercised and held securely with the velcro fastening. More than one band may be applied to any part to obtain greater loading.

It is also possible to join the bands to give a greater length for application to the waist when loading is required for neurologically disabled patients.

Bars and dumbbells The bars from the de Lorme boot can be grasped and used to exercise the muscles of one hand or arm or special dumbbells which are of weights varying from 1 kg to 5 kg may be used.

Barbells These are long bars and heavy weights as used in weight-lifting training. They should be used by reasonably fit patients to strengthen the arms, trunk or legs. It is essential that a clear area of adequate size is in front of the patient before a lift is attempted, that the hands are coated with resin and that the patient knows exactly what to do. The bar may be lifted by the arms with the patient in Lying. It may be lifted using arms and legs (the snatch) with the patient in Walk Crouch, but should not be raised above the head unless the patient is capable of *both* extending the elbows and flexing the shoulders fully as well as thrusting the pelvis forward so that the hips are fully extended to allow the high centre of gravity to fall within the base. The base changes in the course of the lift from Walk to Stride Standing.

CHAPTER 13
Mobilization of Joints

M. HOLLIS

To examine and test a joint prior to mobilization

The medical history should give enough information to allow the therapist to start by observing the patient arriving, undressing both sides of the body and taking up a well-supported position.

Relevant questioning will elicit more information following which the therapist can observe the joint in detail for irregularities, palpate for change of temperature, state of swelling and painful areas.

Testing active range of movement, passive range and resisted range should be followed by accurate recording in accordance with the methods advocated in a book such as 'Joint Motion' (see Bibliography). Tests of muscle power must also be made and recorded.

When the limitation of movement is not due to pathological causes within the joint but to neurological hypertonus then recording of range is irrelevant, but it will be necessary to record the abnormality of the muscle(s) working over the joint.

A joint may be immobile due to three main causes. It may be held still due to protective muscle spasm when severe pain is present. It may be held still and possibly in abnormal posture due to neurological hypertonus (spasticity). It may have little or no range due to pathological causes when changes have taken place to cause shortening of the periarticular soft tissues or bony block as in osteoarthrosis.

Each of these requires a slightly different approach. In the first two cases it is necessary to relieve the spasm by reducing the tone to regain the range. In the case of soft tissue shortening then these structures must be stretched, preferably by the patient. This third group includes those patients who lack the last few degrees of movement due to injury to or surgery upon joints or stiffness due to joints being held still for long periods by fixation.

To relieve painful spasm

The patient is placed in a fully supported position using as large a base as possible. As the patient can often move at another joint and appear to be moving at the painful joint it is frequently necessary to fix joints in which undesirable movement could occur so that 'trick' movements and 'cheating' are prevented. For example, in abduction of one hip unwanted movement in the contralateral hip is prevented by taking the leg to the side of the bed and flexing the knee over the side with the foot supported. Similarly, for extension of the hip unwanted movement is prevented by the patient fully flexing the contralateral leg and, if possible, holding the thigh against the abdomen.

For movement of the glenohumeral joint the patient should be in Crook Lying or Sitting on a seat with a back support to prevent unwanted movement of the lumbar spine. The shoulder girdle is held still by the therapist, so that it is possible to isolate the anatomical movements of abduction and adduction, flexion and extension and medial and lateral rotation.

The best method of stabilizing the patient is by appropriate positioning. The therapist may give further support by using her hands. These methods are better than the use of straps or mechanical devices which should rarely be resorted to. The limb is allowed to rest in its position of minimal pain. If advisable it may be carefully supported in that position by the use of suspension.

The technique of 'Hold Relax' is applied (see Chapter 25) to the muscles which are in protective spasm without allowing any movement to occur at the painful joint, and the technique is repeated until some spasm is relieved and a painfree range of movement becomes possible. It is very important that the movement which is achieved is maintained by the therapist and that repetitive swinging movements of the part are not allowed to take place. In other words, following each relaxation, a little more range is gained and held, and at the end of the treatment the patient will have performed only one movement in that particular direction, but it will have been as full as possible, and the pain-spasm cycle pattern of events will have been broken. If the 'Hold Relax' is applied in suspension it may be necessary and indeed is usually advisable to use the following procedure.

a Obtain a maximum 'Hold' (isotonic contraction of the muscles in spasm).
b Grasp the part with the more distal of the two resisting hands.

c Apply traction and immediately give the command to 'relax' while continuing to increase the traction. The application of traction will prevent the limb from 'leaping' as the muscles relax and is especially essential when suspension is used as the supporting medium and when the muscle action is strong.

Once a range of movement has been achieved then the patient may be asked to perform the required movement actively to come out of the protective spasm position. He is asked to perform a normal movement against the resistance of the therapist thus working the muscles which are antagonistic to those in spasm. In this way these muscles now become the agonists and the muscles which are in spasm become the antagonists and relax reciprocally as reciprocal inhibition is brought about.

At this point in the proceedings the patient may be asked to make frequent active resisted attempts at performing the desired movement at the limit of the available range, while bearing in mind that if a joint has been protected by pain-spasm, there may still be some condition existing at that joint for which too frequently repeated movements are undesirable.

To relieve neurological hypertonus (spasticity)

Although this type of spasm may not be painful, the 'Hold Relax' technique described above may be used. If a little movement is possible, but that movement is limited by the onset of spasticity, then the 'Contract Relax' technique also described in Chapter 25 may be used. Care must be taken that unwanted associated reactions do not occur.

The latter technique may give better results than the 'Hold Relax' technique and when the patient has a controlled movement in the desired direction then Slow Reversals should be given, alternating his movements with the therapist giving maximum resistance to the antagonistic movement and minimum resistance to the muscles which were previously in a spastic state.

In both the above types of loss of movement it may sometimes be necessary to try to obtain irradiation of inhibition. To achieve this the adjacent muscles proximal to the spasm/spasticity are given either resisted movements or isometric contractions in the form of 'Rhythmic Stabilization' (co-contraction of muscles).

This is a particularly useful technique in such conditions as periarthritis of the shoulder when there may be no movement of the glenohumeral joint, but isometric contractions may be given alternately to the various patterns of movement of the scapula (see Chapter 25). They should be followed by 'Hold Relax' to the muscles of the glenohumeral joint which may gain a little range.

Stretching soft tissues which are too tight

This is usually best brought about by the patient attempting to stretch the tissues himself. To this end there are several techniques which may be used. The patient may make repeated efforts at achieving the difficult movement by working the muscles which would bring about the desired movement, e.g. if abduction is limited by tight medial structures the patient works the abductors, or if the last few degrees of elevation of the arm are lost then the patient should make repeated resisted attempts to gain the last few degrees of elevation. The resistance could be given by

the therapist or the patient could push a weight (sandbag) up the wall.

A second technique which may be used is pendular swinging in which the alternations of the pendulum will carry the limb past the limitation of movement and apply repeated minute stretch to the tight structures. The addition of a weight to the end of the limb will both distract the joint surfaces and increase the tendency of the pendulum to swing past the point of limitation. This technique is most commonly used for the shoulder and hip joints, but is equally valuable as a method for the smaller joints such as the wrist and ankle. At these joints rapidly alternating movements are performed and, although the limb of the pendulum is short, the effect of rapid alternations of direction will be to increase momentum in each direction and bring about stretch on tight structures and increase in range. The use of this technique for stiffness of the vertebral region is usually confined to movements of the lumbar spine by swinging the pelvis and legs in suspension thus avoiding dizziness due to alternations in head movement. This is dealt with in Chapter 9.

However, free mobilizing activities for the trunk given in suitable starting positions with the use of the arms to add length to the pendulum may result in a gain in range by the judicious use of self-applied overpressure. Stride Standing trunk side flexion with overpressure, Stretch Stride Standing alternate toe touching with the opposite hand are examples of such exercises and are suitable for selected patients.

A third technique which may be used is that of an auto-pulley circuit (Figures 121 to 123) in which the patient may perform rapid alternations of the two limbs and so carry the stiff joint a little past its limitation each time. Or the patient may apply deliberate slight stretch to the tight structures by an added pull with the contralateral limb.

The fourth technique which is occasionally used is one of self-mobilizing by stretching tight structures using body weight. For example, to stretch a tight tendocalcaneous which is limiting full dorsiflexion of the ankle joint the patient may be put into Step Standing and lean forwards over the bent knee. If both heels are kept on their support the tendocalcaneous is stretched on both legs.

This procedure should NEVER be used unless the muscles acting over the joint being mobilized are already sufficiently strong to maintain the stability of the joint.

Following the relief of spasm or the regaining of range any objective exercises may be used which will increase joint range, while interesting the patient and allowing him to forget his limitations. Some methods of working out such exercises are suggested in Chapter 8 on the use of small apparatus.

CHAPTER 14

Assessment of a Patient's Suitability for Class Treatment

M. HOLLIS & B. SANFORD

All patients should be assessed before being given any treatment but patients are not always assessed as to their suitability for inclusion with a group of people for class work. This omission often arises because the patient is already being treated somewhere other than the gymnasium, e.g. as an inpatient or in an individual therapy room. Such transfers tend to be based on unsuitable standards: a doctor's timetabled prescription; there is a space in the class or there is a waiting list for his individual therapist.

Transfers or admissions to class work should be for positive reasons and should take into consideration all of the following points:

1 Is the patient mentally suitable? In other words can he concentrate, work with others and comprehend and obey commands.

2 Is he physically fit enough to work at the pace of the class? Has he the endurance to carry out exercise for a period of not less than 20 minutes without rests? In other words, are his cardiovascular and respiratory systems normal or will they present complications needing a special class?

3 Can the patient perform all the exercises which form the therapeutic core of the class he is to attend? This means all staff must be familiar with the basic exercises which comprise the penultimate parts of a table, e.g. a patient for the straight leg class must be fully capable of good quadriceps contractions and a patient for a joint mobilizing class must already have an agreed quantity of joint motion and the necessary muscle stability.

4 Is the patient capable of working on his own without close supervision? If there is any doubt two patients with similar disability should be treated together so that the one-to-one relationship is reduced to two-to-one, and each only receives half of the therapist's attention.

5 Has the patient used all or some of the types of equipment which will be used in the class? This means that the therapists must know what sort of exercises are given and what equipment is used in each of the different classes in the gymnasium.

6 Is the patient sufficiently independent to get himself ready for and dressed after a class? This implies not only can he undress and dress the essential areas, but can he balance safely while doing so and possibly also can he walk about without shoes and socks?

7 As class work involves the use of the floor, stools and the fixed apparatus of the gymnasium, the patient must be capable of reaching all of these. Can he, with minimal help, get down on or up from the floor, sit down and stand up and walk the necessary distance?

8 Are there any special social circumstances which would prevent the patient arriving in time for the class? For example the 9.00 a.m. class is not feasible for the one parent who has to see children to school.

To effect the transfer

At the very beginning of the treatment regime the patient should be told that he will have this treatment now and that later, and as he gets better, he will go into a class. He is thus prepared for and accepts class work as an improvement in his own performance. Some patients may need to be reminded at intervals that class work is a goal of good performance and is a progression.

Next he should be introduced to his new therapist and, if possible, be shown at least the room and at best some part of the class he will be joining. He should be advised about special clothing in plenty of time for him to obtain what is needed if it is not provided.

Finally, if necessary, his appointment for any continuing individual treatment should be rearranged and his notes handed on for his new therapist to read before he enters the new sphere of treatment.

CHAPTER 15

Group Exercise

B. SANFORD

In this chapter are suggestions to help the therapist prepare the climate for learning to which every patient is entitled. No one has taught anything until the pupil has learnt something and the degree of success of this communication will determine the satisfaction or otherwise of both teacher and patient. Teaching in a gymnasium presents its own special problems and attention to safety will minimize potential dangers.

SAFETY IN THE GYMNASIUM

All unfamiliar gymnasia should be inspected by the therapist before she prepares a class. The following points should be investigated and possible dangers noted so that exercises can be carried out safely. In the event of the construction of a new gymnasium attempts should be made throughout planning and construction stages to minimize these hazards.

Construction of the gymnasium

Roof Ideally, this should have all the supporting structures enclosed above a flat ceiling. This prevents the unexpected deflection of equipment, e.g. balls, beanbags.

Walls These should be smooth to prevent grazing injuries; and free from unnecessary protruding structures, e.g. clocks should be recessed and covered with wire mesh and mirrors should fold and reverse to form a flush surface when not in use. Unavoidable protrusions should be carefully situated. A semi-gloss paint will reduce glare from the sun on those walls likely to be affected.

Floor This should be constructed of suitable wooden laths running across the room. This type of floor gives some spring and the direction of the laths being opposite to that of the general movement reduces slipperiness. The floor should be cleaned in accordance with the builder's instructions and at no time should polish be applied.

Windows These should be sufficient to provide adequate lighting with opening elements enough to secure reasonable ventilation. They are best situated well above the level of activity to prevent draughts on patients when they are opened to avoid a sleepy or unsavoury atmosphere. Protection from breakage by moving balls, etc., is also effected by high positioning. The incorporation of mesh-integrated glass is a good safeguard against injury from falling glass.

Lighting Artificial lights should be adequate in number and spacing. They should not cast shadows and should be protected from the danger of moving small equipment. They are

141

best built flush with the ceiling, and protected by mesh-integrated glass.

Heating   The heating system should be unobtrusive but adequate for the size of the room. Hot air entering the room through adjustable grids seems to be the most practical solution and unavoidable radiators should be protected. A stuffy and therefore dangerously sleepy atmosphere should be avoided by using a thermostat.

Apparatus in the gymnasium

Fixed apparatus should be installed by experts and regular checks should take place (in accordance with the safety regulations of the DHSS). Obvious faults should be dealt with immediately and such apparatus put out of use. Moveable apparatus, large and small, should be stored neatly in an easily accessible adjoining area, which allows simultaneously free entry and exit of a reasonably large number of people. Agility apparatus should be moved with care, and patients should not use it until it has been checked for safety in its new position by the therapist. Small equipment should be moved about in suitable containers and not left lying around on the gymnasium floor whilst exercises are in progress. Apparatus involved in an accident should be retained for inspection.

PEOPLE IN THE GYMNASIUM

These include patients and therapists.

Punctuality   The therapist should already be in the gymnasium when the first patient enters. A full period of treatment is important to all patients and they may well start their own exercises using equipment which could be dangerous. Patients, too, should arrive punctually so as not to miss the early part of the class intended to prepare them and to produce a good circulatory effect for safe, stronger exercises later.

Dress   This should be such as to allow safe, free movement, e.g. shorts for a knee class, a sleeveless garment for a hand class. The therapist should be easily distinguished by a uniform outfit. If worn, the footwear of both patients and therapists should be lightweight with non-slip soles, and under no circumstances should socks or tights only be allowed. If hair is long, it should be suitably tied back and well secured so as not to swing. Watches, jewellery, etc., should be removed to prevent scratching injuries. These last points apply to both patient and therapist.

Other factors

The number of patients in any one class should not exceed eight to twelve (according to type of class) and the therapist should know every patient by name. There is a special danger in teaching anonymous patients; they cannot be prevented from individual hazards. Similarly, the therapist should be sure the patients know her name. Of primary importance is the firm mastering of the word STOP. It ensures a quick control of a foreseeable accident. It is essential too that not only is each patient's diagnosis known, but also any other relevant medical factors, e.g. heart condition, deafness, etc. Finally, the therapist should know and apply all the basic rules of teaching (see later).

If, despite all reasonable care and attention to inherent dangers, an accident occurs deal with it calmly and competently, then report the details in writing immediately to the appropriate department.

GENERAL TEACHING TECHNIQUE

It is often claimed that good teachers are born, not made. This is not so, only some good teachers are born and many more are created by determination and deep understanding between staff and student. Apprehension is an essential ingredient of good teaching and the fact that initially it often displays itself as a deep fear should be accepted as normal. Time and actual teaching practice expertly guided can put this to good advantage. It should be remembered that to the injured exercise is not a reflex physical process, and it is necessary to stimulate the desire to perform. Only by complete involvement on the part of the teacher will this be successful. The following basic rules should be observed.

Teach firmly and positively but not aggressively. Tell the patients what to do, rather than ask them. 'Please' and 'can you' should initially form no part of the command. It is not easy and often feels rude and abrupt not to use these phrases in the early stages of learning to take a class. Patients who are often frightened and in pain should be given no hint that they may fail to perform what they are asked to do. To help achieve this the best use of the teacher's voice should be regarded as of extreme importance.

Voice

The correct use of the voice is an important factor in ensuring the success of the class. It should be stimulating, portray enthusiasm and enjoyment, whilst working at least as hard and keenly as the patient's muscles. The most carefully planned class may be rendered ineffective by poor vocal delivery.

Patients best hear sounds which come from their front or sides, and the therapist should bear this in mind when it is necessary to change her own position, or that of the patients, e.g. when patients roll over from Lying to Prone Lying the therapist should move to the opposite end of the class. The voice should always be firm and audible, have clear diction and a variety of intonation. Words should be carefully separated and not allowed to run into each other. Particular care is needed at the end of the first word when the same consonant ends one word and starts the next, e.g. '*let your leg go forward*', or when any two hard consonants come together, e.g. '*sit down*'. The volume should vary to suit the size, nature and participants in the class. A rehabilitation group of boisterous young people will require greater volume than a group of geriatric ladies. When working in the open air a greater volume will be needed due to the lack of throwback from walls.

The voice will be most clearly heard if the muscles of the neck, shoulder and shoulder girdle are relaxed and an effort is made to feel that the words come from the abdomen. Daily practice of deep breathing will help, making a long 'ah' sound in expiration. In this way deeper, more audible tones will be produced and the therapist will be spared a perpetual sore throat. If the size of the class is large the therapist should feel that her voice is thrown high to the back of the room.

How a movement is to be performed should be indicated by the therapist's voice. She may wish it to be done quickly or slowly and the speed of her voice should vary accordingly. Movements requiring prolonged effort should be helped by corresponding effort on appropriate words in the therapist's voice. When encouraging a patient to lift a heavy weight, the word '*lift*' should be prolonged and have a rising inflexion. When helping a patient to relax a limb, the therapist may use the word '*drop*', which should be sudden and have a falling inflexion. Movements to be performed lightly need a lighter tone. Words should be produced in a staccato manner for light, tripping movements.

Variety in the choice of words used is stimulating, but care must be taken to avoid the use of technical terms, e.g. '*bend*' not '*flex*', '*turn*' not '*rotate*'. Some knowledge of local words and phrases could be an asset, but should not be overused. Monotony will be avoided if important words are emphasized, usually verbs, adverbs or adjectives, e.g. '*PUSH* your partner over'; 'throw the ball *HIGH* into the air'; 'make your jump *LONG*'.

The successful use of the voice will only be achieved if the therapist is completely convinced of the effectiveness of the exercises she is presenting. Careful preparation of all exercises is essential (see p. 147).

Positioning

Within reason, use all available space. The positioning of both patients and therapist should be such that observation of expected difficulties is easy. Movement of the therapist, any part of a patient or of apparatus should not present danger to anyone in the room. If the sun is shining into the room, place the patients with their backs to it; the therapist's position can be adapted more easily to a safe position in the shade. Patients likely to need extra help should be at the sides of the class, so that as it is given, the therapist can, at all times, have the whole class in view. If using a circular formation the therapist should teach from the outside so that no patient is ever behind her.

Patients who have special problems, e.g. the deaf or blind should be positioned where they can most benefit from the group. The deaf may be able to lip read and the blind will need to hear well, so they should be near the therapist.

Teaching an exercise

All exercises used in teaching should be within the experience of the therapist. This does not necessarily mean that she must be able to give a perfect demonstration, but that she is at least aware of potential difficulties. There are four clear stages in teaching an exercise.

Starting position   This should be carefully chosen for each exercise bearing in mind what the therapist is trying to achieve. That it is correct is of utmost importance. If it is wrong then any movement from it will inevitably be performed inefficiently and uneconomically. A starting position used for successive exercises should be checked before proceeding, and all starting positions should be observed continuously.

The exercise to be performed   This can be taught by words and demonstration or by a combination of both. Words should be clear, brief, to the point and above all audible, bearing in mind that several classes and individual treatments may be in progress at the same time. Tell the patients what to do, and get the exercise going as quickly as possible, remembering that ears 'shut off' fairly quickly. Demonstration can be of assistance in teaching those exercises which otherwise would necessitate lengthy explanations, but bear in mind that a full day's teaching in a gymnasium can be very strenuous—choose the demonstrations wisely. If this method of teaching is used, the exercise should be performed without fault and from a position (or series of positions) from which every patient can see.

Help, advice and encouragement should be given as the exercise is in progress with a view to improving performance (see section on observation and correction).

The termination The exercise should finally be brought to a close when the therapist feels that the time is appropriate, and not when the patient feels like it. This should normally be when a further continuance of the exercise would result in reduced performance.

Observation and correction

This calls for tact and initiative. Always teach to avoid the necessity to correct. The need for too much correction indicates lack of care in preparation. A dynamic standing position is normally most suitable from which to observe faults. Teaching in other positions should be reserved for special occasions, e.g. if helping a patient or teaching children (see Chapter 18). If it is necessary to use other positions for demonstrating an exercise, return to the standing position as soon as possible. A teacher should change her position in relation to the class according to the faults an exercise is likely to present, but any movement should be for a purpose, and not just a continuous irritating pace backwards and forwards.

Observation should be done systematically from side to side or front to back and the therapist should spend time learning to make full use of all her peripheral vision. This is easily done by fixing her eyes on any stationary object and increasing her awareness of other movement in the room. In the first instance, correction should be of the whole class. The therapist should pick out the more widespread mistakes and correct positively by encouragement and help as the exercise is in progress. Care must be taken to deal with one fault at a time, not forgetting the starting position. Individual corrections must be dealt with very tactfully in a class, and all improvement, not necessarily perfection, should be suitably rewarded with praise—remember success breeds success. The patient should always feel that the therapist's standard is high, but individual effort should not go unrewarded. Should all effort to correct an exercise fail—stop the class and reteach, if necessary breaking the exercise down into fewer components.

General points

It is important that groups are used for the benefit of patients and not because of a staff shortage. All patients should have had at least one individual treatment for assessment or teaching purposes and should have been selected for group work by the therapist in the gymnasium in consultation with other appropriate staff (see Chapter 14). It is essential to know the patient's previous and future intended occupation so as to have an idea of earlier fitness and strength and to be able to gear the treatment to that needed for the future.

The cooperation of the patient is vital. All successful teaching is based on this mutual trust both in the class and in the daily practice of exercises to be done at home (see Chapter 16). All exercises should be carefully chosen and suited to the age and sex of the patient. They should show variety, sometimes stimulating, sometimes quietening, perhaps rhythmic or to command, formal or informal. Every physical activity, e.g. entering or leaving the gymnasium, collecting and clearing away apparatus, should be used for teaching purposes. These activities give a useful knowledge of a person's independence away from the hospital and can provide natural breaks between physically exhausting exercises.

Should the therapist herself feel bored with the class then undoubtedly the patients will feel likewise. Boredom arises because she is not completely involved in making the exercises enjoyable, and from total involvement alone comes the satisfaction of a job well done.

MIXED ABILITY GROUPS

These can be useful when there are small numbers of patients at different stages of recovery from similar disabilities, for whom group treatment would be beneficial. A typical class in the younger age group could consist of patients all of whom are at different stages of recovery from knee surgery or injury. In the older age group hemiplegics or amputees could each form satisfactory classes. To prevent too much movement of patients, the room should be arranged so that apparatus needed for similar disabilities is adjacent. For example, patients with hand injuries or handling problems will need both tables and

adjacent small apparatus, while those with balance problems will need to be near both parallel bars and stools.

Exercises from which all patients benefit should be taken at the beginning of the class and also a group activity for all at the end if time permits. For these collective exercises the patients should be positioned so that those needing extra help are together where the therapist can give help whilst watching the rest of the group. Some may need only a little help and can often be interspersed with the more advanced patients who will benefit from giving a little aid to the less able.

The middle of the treatment session should consist of exercises designed for specific disabilities and the patients should be repositioned in the appropriate area and possibly with the designated apparatus. At this stage they each may be performing a different exercise and the therapist should be constantly alert and ready to move to prevent dangerous situations developing or to improve a patient's performance. These exercises should be of a more functional nature and the patient should easily be able to move to another task if the room is correctly planned. Mixed ability groups inevitably need more time than groups of patients with more equal ability and should not be attempted unless at least an hour's treatment time is available.

CHAPTER 16
Preparation of Classes

B. SANFORD

Confidence is the keynote to successful teaching and, for this reason, the therapist should never teach an unprepared class. If unavoidable circumstances make prior warning impossible, it is best to let the patients practise home exercises for a few minutes as she quickly works out a suitable series of exercises. It is never satisfactory for a therapist to be thinking of the second exercise as she is teaching the first.

It is necessary to make two types of preparation for class work.

Scheme of treatment

This should be a plan of treatment including all the aims of a particular series of classes, and the methods and types of exercises to be used to achieve these. At all times, a scheme of treatment must be aimed at enabling the patient to live the fullest possible life which his immediate problems will allow. Therefore, treatment of any particular part must be related to the body as a whole. Each scheme should cover the period of time from the patient joining the class, to the time of his progression to a more advanced class or to discharge. Should it be concerned with the class prior to his discharge, it should invariably lead to sufficient recovery for the patient to return to his chosen occupation.

Table of exercises

This should consist of a series of suitable exercises to be taught during any one period of treatment, and should be based on the scheme of treatment previously worked out. The therapist should include at least one exercise for each aim with a second or third exercise for the more important ones. All exercises should be prepared with function in mind, and care should be taken not to fatigue individual muscle groups by using the same ones in consecutive exercises. When the therapist is taking several classes in succession, it is advisable for her to have quick reminders of the order of exercises on easily accessible cards.

All classes should show a similar pattern, and for an allocation of a 30-minute period in the gymnasium, 20 minutes of exercise should be possible (allowing for undressing and dressing). An average of ten exercises will be needed for this period.

1 An introductory exercise which should have a 'warming up' effect on appropriate areas. This should allow great freedom of movement, and unless injuries make it impossible, it is best taken in a standing position. It should involve movement of a large joint or joints related to the actual area of concern, e.g. in a hand class an exercise involving shoulder movement would be suitable. If the

147

class is concerned equally with the whole body, then an exercise involving large movements of the whole body is appropriate, e.g. an easy game previously taught.

2 This should be followed by three or four exercises which localize movement if this is appropriate, and starting positions should be carefully chosen. If restricted movement is no longer a problem, the exercises in this section should not demand precision or too much strength; the body must work up to these. In a general class large movements of the trunk, legs and arms are suitable, and, when dealing with more specific areas, the larger muscle groups should be used.

3 The patients should now be ready for exercises demanding range of movement, greater strength, and/or precision, taken in the more dynamic positions of everyday life. These should include exercises involving quick movement and quick thinking. As the patients progress, the number of less specific exercises (as in 2 above) should be reduced and be replaced by more in this group.

4 The climax of the class should consist of a game or activities involving all the skills which have been taught, and if possible involving the interaction of all the members of the group.

5 The class should end on a quiet note with appropriate postural advice. This is a convenient time to deal with individual posture problems of everyday life.

The original table of exercises should be recorded and progressed systematically each day. One or two well-performed exercises may be changed at each treatment, so that a good part of the class always remains familiar to the patients. In this way the whole table of exercises will eventually be progressed and boredom prevented. The therapist should at all times make sure that the progressions are within the scope of the patients or she may well find they 'give up'. Finally, any prepared exercises which, through lack of time are omitted, should certainly be included in the next treatment.

Progression of exercise

Carefully planned progression will ensure that the injured part of the body returns to the highest possible degree of function in the shortest possible time. Such progression can be judged to be successful when the injured area, having been worked to the point of fatigue in any one treatment session, recovers so as to enable the patient to take part fully in the next. Most progressions can, and should if necessary, be tailored to accommodate individual members of each group. Only the observation of the therapist in charge can decide which type of progression is relevant and when this should be implemented. Constant reference to the original scheme of exercises will serve as a guide.

Starting positions Progression is effected by changing the starting position so as to alter the effect gravity has on a muscle action when performing a movement. If gravity is counterbalanced, muscle work is easier than if gravity is resisting a movement, e.g. if a patient is lying on the floor lifting his arms sideways, the abductors of the shoulder will work less hard than if he is performing the same exercise sitting on a stool.

Change in the size of the base provided by a starting position alters the degree of difficulty of an exercise. A broad base, e.g. Stride Standing or Walk Standing gives greater stability to a movement than a small base, e.g. Close Standing or Toe Standing. An exercise performed on a stationary surface is easier than the same exercise performed on a moveable surface because of the extra balance involved in the latter, e.g. bouncing a ball with the feet on a balance board is harder than bouncing a ball with the feet on the floor.

Endurance There should be a gradual increase in the length of time spent performing each exercise. This may be controlled by measured time or by counting the number of repetitions, whichever is appropriate. The ultimate goal should be within the limits of the patient's ability and concentration. Endless repetitions of simple exercises may cause regression through loss of interest. The total duration of each session should be increased gradually. For instance, a new patient may get maximum benefit from just 20 minutes daily exercise. This can be increased to 30 minutes, then to 45 minutes and eventually to an hour or a full day's treatment. This will depend on the needs of the patient and the life style he is to resume. As the treatment time increases the therapist should ensure that exercises putting excessive stress on the cardiovascular and respiratory systems do not follow in rapid succession. In this way complete rest periods will be kept to a minimum.

Muscle loading (See Chapter 12.) Sandbags provide a useful and cheap means of muscle loading in group work and are most frequently used in the re-education of limbs. They can be used to resist both isometric and isotonic muscle work. Using considered judgement the therapist should introduce weights in appropriate exercises to offer resistance in addition to that of the weight of the limb. Without added resistance such exercises would need an unacceptable number of repetitions in order for the muscle to reach momentary

exhaustion. Loading can be progressed according to the needs of the individual. An example of a suitable exercise is Backward Prop Support Long Sitting, straight leg lifting and lowering. Weight bearing exercises for suitable lower limb injuries should be progressed alongside muscle loading and should replace it completely in the later stages of recovery. Lower limb joints are normally subjected to compression and to encourage normal functioning weight bearing exercises must be introduced as soon as possible. In addition muscles should be re-educated to work in a functional capacity.

Levers (See Chapter 3.) A short weight arm is more easily moved than a long one and exercises can be progressed using this principle. For example when working the back extensor muscles in Prone Lying, head and shoulder lifting, at first the arms should remain at the sides of the body. The exercise can be made harder by stretching the arms out in front to make the lever longer. If the starting position is changed to Across Prone Lying (form) the lever is lengthened because the fulcrum is moved from the chest to the pelvis.

Range (See Chapter 1.) Muscles work most easily in their middle range and this is in many cases the range in which they produce functional movements. Weak muscles should be re-educated first of all in this range, progressing to the more difficult inner and outer ranges. Strengthening of muscles which control range should precede increase in joint range or control may be inefficient, e.g. if the knee joint has mobility without muscle strength the leg will collapse on weight bearing.

Speed Alteration in the speed of an exercise

is a useful means of progression. The speed may need to be increased or decreased to effect the desired progression. Walking may become harder if done more slowly because of the harder balance involved. Throwing a ball against a wall and catching it again becomes more difficult when done more quickly. This demands better coordination and speedier muscle actions.

The therapist should allow a gradually shorter time for changing from one starting position to another and for collecting and putting away apparatus. The patient should be encouraged to dress and undress at greater speed. In industry today, piece work on production lines makes the time taken to do a job of paramount importance.

The condition of the patient should be checked at each session. Any signs of regression should be investigated. Should pain, swelling, reddening of the skin, reduced ability to exercise be present, progressions in exercises introduced at the previous session should be omitted.

HOME EXERCISES

In order for treatment to be fully effective, exercises carefully selected from those taught in the class should be practised daily at home. It is not always easy for patients who are working full time to set aside special periods for exercise during the day and for such people some of the exercises chosen should be able to be practised at work, e.g. an office worker with a knee injury could practise isotonic quadriceps exercises under his desk, or perhaps he could walk to and from work.

All home exercises should have been taught very thoroughly and the therapist must be satisfied that the patient can perform them

unsupervised. As each exercise selected for home practice is introduced, suggestions for recognizing improvement should be given to the patient, e.g. improvement in shoulder movement could be measured against the good arm with the help of a mirror. Improvement in errors of gait can be recognized with the aid of a mirror and improvement in muscle endurance can be measured by noting the length of time for which an exercise can be performed. Alternatively the number of repetitions of the exercise may be counted. The therapist should bear in mind that in modern houses, rooms are small and ceilings are low so the exercises should not need height, large areas of uninterrupted floor space or involve quick movement of dangerous apparatus, e.g. exercises involved running or high throwing of balls should be avoided.

Patients who are at home should be encouraged to practise their exercises for short periods throughout the day. A 15–20-minute exercise period at the beginning of the day when the body has been resting is advisable with further 10-minute periods spread throughout the day, e.g. mid-morning, lunchtime, mid-afternoon and in the evening. In the early stages of treatment when muscles are very weak, exercise periods could be shorter and taken more often, and in the later stages effort should be made to increase the time spent at each practice session. It is advisable for patients to stick to their routine unless special circumstances make this impossible. Fatigue due to inadequate rest periods can make the exercises less effective. Patients who are working all day should make time for 15–20 minutes concentrated practice in the morning and in the evening.

Exercises practised at home should be checked regularly by the therapist and progress recorded. The patient should be told in what order the exercises should be practised and how many times to repeat each one, the latter being progressed as the patient improves. Circuit routines are particularly suitable for more advanced patients (see Chapter 12). If small equipment is to be used it should be cheap to buy, e.g. a small ball, or be such that may be represented by objects found in the home, e.g. a rolling pin or a rolled up newspaper can be used instead of a pole and weights for resistance can be made up of packs of household goods, etc.

In addition to practising exercises taught in the class, many daily activities serve as 'home exercises'. A shoulder may be exercised by a housewife each time she cleans a window if she is instructed to clean as large an area as possible before moving her feet to a new position. If she stands in a position giving a large base (e.g. Stride Standing) a large range of shoulder movement will be achieved. Postnatal exercises particularly should be incorporated into the mother's very busy new routine at home, e.g. trunk rotation may be practised when ironing if she collects the clothes from one side and puts them away at the other, provided she keeps her feet still.

The therapist should realize that patients are full of human failings and exercising at home will be conveniently forgotten unless the therapist is conscientious in checking progress each time the patient attends for treatment. Only by continuous effort both at home and at the treatment session can the patient expect a satisfactory recovery.

CHAPTER 17
Competition: Sport in Medicine

M. HOLLIS & B. SANFORD

Competition is an inherent part of all active exercise therapy, and group work presents a variety of opportunities for its use. It is stimulating and helps patients to forget their disabilities. Each individual in the group should be encouraged to compete against his own weaknesses by working towards appropriate goals set by the therapist. Working *with* a partner is particularly suitable for a class with a reasonably wide range of abilities, provided care is exercised in sorting out partners. Competition is unconsciously stimulated in their effort to help each other. Working *against* a partner may also be used, perhaps competing to see which patient can perform a series of movements most quickly, or for the longest period of time, e.g. skipping in a leg class.

Competitive table games may be used successfully for re-educating patients who require manipulative skills or coordination between hand and eye. Many suitable games are marketed, e.g. draughts, tiddley-winks, dominoes and various card games. These can be adapted by the therapist to suit the need, e.g. tiddley-winks may be flicked on to a large lid if the patients have insufficient control to aim into a small cup, and draughts may be played with pieces of 'Lego' which give resistance when 'crowning' the counters, if this is required for the pincer grip.

Competitive team games may be of two types; 'minor' games in which several small

teams compete against each other or 'major' games in which two large teams compete. Most 'major' and 'minor' games are easily adapted for use either indoors or outdoors. In a 'minor' game, each member of a team has to perform in turn the same activity or series of activities and the winning team is the one to finish first, e.g. a variety of appropriate objects may be passed along a line of patients re-educating their hands to the movements of objects along a production line. The team taking the least time is the winner.

'Major' games include games such as volley ball, netball or basketball, various types of rounders, etc. In both 'major' or 'minor' games care must be taken to avoid leaving patients inactive for any length of time. The rules of all games should be to ensure safety and enjoyment and in remedial work may have to be adapted to suit the patient's needs.

It is important to start playing the game as quickly as possible, and instructions should be clear and concise. The following pattern for teaching is successful.

1 Select the teams of equal strength as far as is possible and put the players roughly into position for play, e.g. for volley ball place one team on each side of the net, as this will help the explanation of the game. If playing outside, keep the patients within hearing distance.

2 Explain briefly what each team has to do introducing as few rules as possible to make the game safe and enjoyable.
3 Play the game for a short trial period and use this time to clear up errors and note any instructions that have been misunderstood. Stop the game and answer individual queries.
4 Restart the game and either act as umpire yourself or appoint someone to do this.
5 Make sure you give a result at the end.

Whilst the game is in progress the therapist should give help and encouragement, particularly to the weaker team, and good or improved play should be commented upon. Varied rules can be applied if these seem necessary to suit the progress of the patients, e.g. in volley ball the normal rule allows three passes on one side of the net before the ball must pass over the net. The author finds this rule restricting and varies or omits its application when patients with limited speed and skill are playing. In this way patients will be allowed to have a sense of achievement and perhaps to reach a personal goal. At all times competition must be fair. Unfairness leads to frustration, disinterest, danger from frayed tempers and results in lack of progress by the patient.

SPORT IN MEDICINE

The value of all forms of sporting activity for those who are physically disabled, whether temporarily or permanently, cannot be overestimated.

Solo ventures such as learning to swim or to ride, or competitive activities such as table tennis or netball offer recreation, the opportunity to be normal in a different environment and social contact with resultant uplift in psychological morale.

To the temporarily handicapped the opportunity to use an old recreational sport or adopt a new one offers a stimulus to the hope of recovery and will also speed up the recovery rate by increasing endurance, strength and coordination.

To the more permanently handicapped who have from birth led a limited and restricted life, sporting facilities now available to them offer new dimensions of living. The joy of seeing a paralysed child swim well using his arms alone or even only small movements of his hands is an experience well worth the time and effort spent in organizing the teaching of such a feat.

Riding is another solo sport which has given handicapped people, whether their handicap be congenital or acquired, an opportunity to learn and enjoy an activity so much enjoyed by many young people of normal physique. It is especially useful in teaching balance in a new dimension and release from the confines of a wheelchair, and from the fear of falling often relieves many of the symptoms.

Competitive sport such as that organized by many rehabilitation units and for the Parolympics has meant a worldwide increase in the care and attention given to those confined to a wheelchair. Arising originally from the work of Sir Ludwig Guttmann and his team at Stoke Mandeville Hospital, sport for the disabled has come to mean competitive swimming, archery, table tennis, javelin throwing, netball, putting the shot and others.

The list of available activities grows as the interest of more and more people is captured and rules are adapted for the particular ability and disability. It may be that many handicapped people can compete on equal terms with the able bodied. Deafness, for example, is no deterrent in many sporting activities and blind people also have their adapted equipment.

At the same time as we concern ourselves with the more dramatic events such as spinal injury, it must not be forgotten that a swimming pool may for example be the only place where a rigid sufferer from ankylosing spondylitis can be free from pain, and, by doing a minimal arm movement can propel himself through the water.

The teaching of each sport and the rules for each game require extensive investigation; the present names of Secretaries and addresses of the various organizations who can supply further information are given:

The Sports Council, 70 Brompton Road, London SW3 1EX.

The Scottish Sports Council, 1 St Colme Street, Edinburgh EH3 6AA.

British Sports Association for the Disabled (BSAD), Ludwig Guttmann Sports Centre for the Disabled, Harvey Road, Aylesbury, Buckinghamshire HP21 8PP

Institute of Sports Medicine, Ling House, 10 Nottingham Place, London W1M 4AX.

Riding for the Disabled Association, National Agricultural Centre, Kenilworth, Warwickshire CV8 2LR.

CHAPTER 18
Exercises for Babies and Children

M. HOLLIS & B. SANFORD

The smallest and most immature baby which is fit to be handled can be exercised in a routine in sequence and will eventually participate in the routine performing active assisted movements.

The baby should be completely undressed and laid on a firm but well padded surface, covered with a washable terry towelling sheet. This is a surface with a reasonably high co-efficient of friction. Initially the baby should lie supine with the feet towards the therapist who should talk all the time to the child giving the same commands in the same tone during each performance of the exercise, so that the baby learns to associate the same sound with the same movement, thus learning with the ears and proprioceptive mechanism together. Start with the larger joints of the limbs. A suitable routine would be:

To grasp the ankles (Figure 144) and first slowly then quickly flex and extend the knees and hips within the available range.

Two slow movements with each leg can be followed by three to four quick movements.

Next the legs are straightened at the knee, though in a very young baby it will not be feasible to straighten the hips, and they must not be forced, and the legs are then abducted and adducted.

This can be followed by individual movements to each ankle joint in turn, plantar and dorsiflexion.

Then the baby's feet are held with the knees and hips partly flexed (Figure 145) and pressure is applied with the thumb on the plantar surface of the area of the metatarsophalangeal joints. The response will be

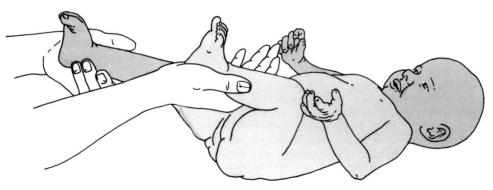

Figure 144 Flexion and extension of the hips and knees within the available range.

155

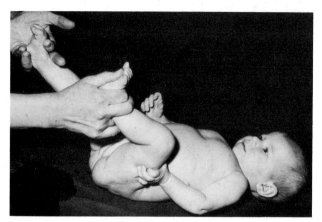

Figure 145 Flexion of the left toes in response to thumb pressure. The right toes are extending.

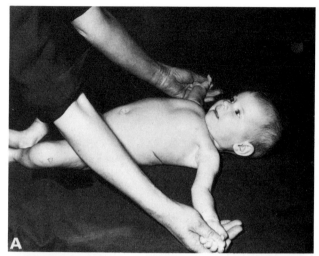

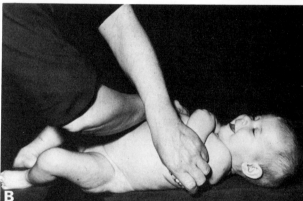

Figure 146 A, The grasp for abduction of the arms; B, Flexion of the arms.

plantarflexion of the toes. Removal of the pressure will produce extension of the toes shortly afterwards.

If it is desired to produce active contraction of individual muscles or muscle groups the muscle belly should be stroked, usually from proximal to distal, e.g. a sharp stroke over the peronei will cause the foot to be actively everted, and dorsiflexion can be produced by stroking over the anterior tibials. After three to four strokes the response dies away.

The attention is now turned to the arms. The therapist's thumbs are placed on the baby's palms and her hands grasp his forearms (Figure 146). Movements again start at the larger joints.

Flex the arms across the chest and extend them in abduction. Some elbow movement will also occur (Cabmans swing). When this movement is performed care must be taken to avoid compression of the chest and each arm takes its turn to be the upper arm. The arms can then be circled, though in younger babies the amount of elevation will be limited (Figure 147).

With the elbow flexed the forearm can be pronated and supinated, and by removing the therapist's fingers from grasping the baby's forearms it is possible to perform flexion and extension of the wrist and hand. This is easier if the baby still retains the grasp reflex.

Trunk exercises can follow and the baby should have the hips and knees bent so that the legs are held in the Crook Lying position with one hand, of which the forefinger is between the ankles (Figure 148) and the other hand is inserted under the sacrum to tickle in order the sacral, lumbar and thoracic regions producing an extensor response—a pelvic raise and arching in each part of the back in turn.

Retaining the same grip on the feet with one hand, the baby is presented with the ring and forefinger of the other hand to grasp. The therapist grasps the baby's wrists with her thumb and little finger and keeps the wrists apart with the middle finger so holding the arms comfortably together in mid-line (Figure 149). Then by pulling gently on the arms and shoulder girdle the baby will be persuaded to attempt a head raise. Only a young neonate, a disabled or very weak baby, will have a total head lag. The pull on the arms lifts the chest slightly, stretches the anterior neck muscles which twitch in response and after a few treatments most babies show diminished head lag.

Next the baby should be turned to the Prone position by retaining the same grip, but by straightening the legs and releasing one of his hands to roll him gently towards the free hand and so into Prone. Very young babies (under 6 weeks old) will lie with flexed hips and knees. A gentle pull on the feet held as before with the forefinger extended up between the ankles at the same time as the back is tickled in each area in turn will result in a head raise and even an attempted back extension.

Still retaining the same grasp on the feet and placing one hand under the upper abdomen, the baby is picked up and a gentle pull is exerted on the legs (Figure 150). This produces an even more effective head raise. Flexion of hips and knees will produce flexion of the trunk again.

The baby is replaced on the support and turned back into the Lying position ready to be

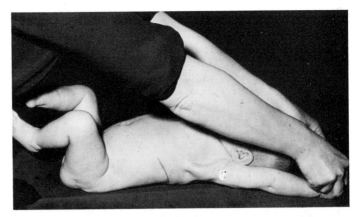

Figure 147   Elevation of the arms.

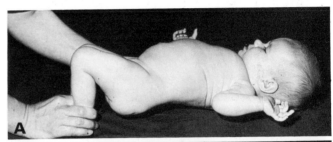

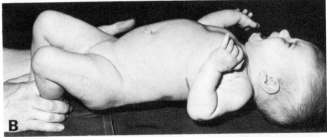

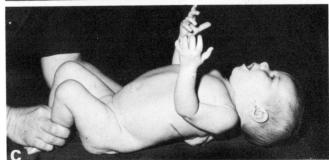

Figure 148   A, Pelvis raise; B, Lumbar spine arch; C, Thoracic spine arch. NOTE: The grasp on the feet and ankles.

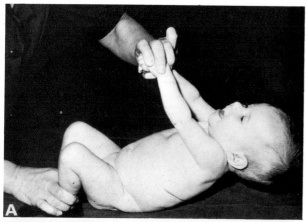

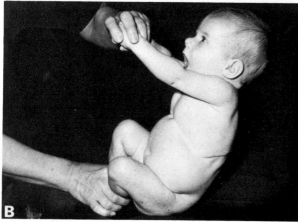

Figure 149   The grasp to assist: A, head and shoulder flexion; B, sitting up.

picked up by his feet. The therapist places the forefinger of each hand across the metatarsophalangeal joints and grasps with her thumb and remaining fingers round the ankles. She then slowly raises the legs, buttocks, back and head free from the support and moves away from it, so that she can hold the child easily in free space in which he can move. Gentle alternate forward and backward movement of the

legs as in a walking pattern will cause the upper trunk to rotate. Moving the left leg forward and right leg back causes the baby to rotate to his own left. Gentle lateral swinging may be performed or alternatively one leg can be bent at the hip and knee and he will side flex his trunk towards that leg (Figures 151 and 152). When the baby is put down he is first raised well above the support, lowered until his head just touches it and quickly rolled down onto his back and pelvis.

If, throughout this routine of exercises, a smooth continuity of movement is maintained with a 'sing song' sequence of commands or names of actions, the baby will quickly learn the routine. This routine should be followed every time the baby is treated and is entirely suitable for babies who through sickness in their early months are physically backward, or for babies who have been socially and emotionally deprived and are in consequence physically unstimulated. The routine may also be performed on babies who have congenital physical abnormalities which involve prolonged fixation, e.g. club feet. The routine also has value for babies who are born with injuries such as fractures and Erb's palsy or torticollis. It has a place in the treatment of premature babies.

In this routine the therapist is using the stretch reflex to induce the baby to active contraction whether by performing passive movements or stroking over muscles. It has been the author's experience that all babies respond well to this routine and learn it within 3 weeks and are physically stronger within that period of time. It is not a routine suitable for babies with neurological disorders such as cerebral palsy, but useful for those who are mentally subnormal. Babies who are physically backward catch up more quickly to normal responses following the application of the routine. It is a suitable regime to teach a mother to perform at home, but should be abandoned when the child is physically normal for his age. Suspension by the feet should not be given to heavy babies and may be the first part of the regime to be abandoned.

INFANTS

The term infant is applied to those capable of understanding play and vocal encouragement. A wide selection of toys is now available for the therapist to use for play/exercise for this age group.

It should be remembered that one can engage the attention of small children for only very short periods of time, i.e. the concentration span is shortest in the young and therefore a great variety of simple or ingenious exercises must be thought up. All exercises should be applied with the aims of treatment in mind.

Only three or four repetitions may be possible with very young infants, but some children like endless repetitions. A large selection of toys should not be displayed at one time but most of them kept out of sight until they are needed. The treatment should be given in the smallest available space remembering that to an infant big spaces are infinite and probably frightening. It may be better initially to play with a well-loved toy which the child may be using as an emotional prop for the temporary deprivation of his mother and normal environment.

In giving exercises to small children it is important to remember that ill health or distress reduces the mental age and he should not be expected to perform at his normal age level even though the child is known to be socially, emotionally and mentally normal.

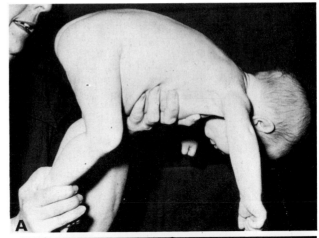

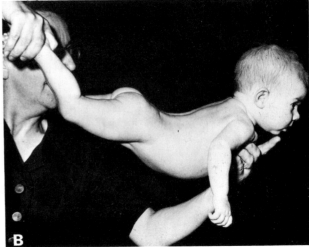

Figure 150 A, Supported ready for arching; B, A gentle pull on the legs of this 6-month-old baby produces a good head and back extension.

This is very evident in a ward of sick children when normally independent children become either attention seeking or withdrawn due to the change of environment as well as ill health.

Most activities can be performed as a game, to nursery rhymes or rhyming songs. Skilled

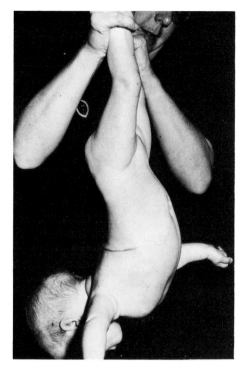

Figure 151   Foot support trunk rotation.

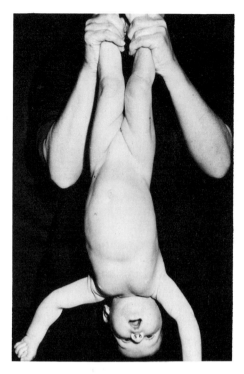

Figure 152   Foot support left leg flexion with left trunk flexion.

musical performance is not demanded, but lively vocal stimulation will usually produce a satisfactory performance when it is performed with enjoyment on the part of the therapist and the child's attention is still commanded. The moment the child's attention wanders a different exercise and a different song or rhyme pattern should be substituted and even a change of exercise to another part of the body. So long as there is constant return to the part that needs most work there is no harm in diversion. The same person should give the exercises at every visit if possible so that the infant feels secure in this social contact. The child should be encouraged and praised for each success.

It is easy to forget that children will become exhausted by effort and concentration, but that they will express fatigue differently from an adult. A fall off in performance, an increase in irritability or a refusal to perform at all will signal that it is time to go away for the time being and return later in the day. Always give the child something to do or he will find it for himself and may do neither the therapist's exercises nor his own.

For this group and those in the next age group the clothing of the therapist may be important. Again hugeness is suggested by a person wearing all the same colour.

OLDER CHILDREN

As children get older they often like to exhibit their skills especially to the parent who, unless they interfere in the treatment, should be encouraged to stay in the room. Mothers and fathers should be discouraged from resigning their parental role in the interests of becoming full time therapists in order to 'push' the physical progress of their child to a daily limit. Nevertheless, an understanding parent who can encourage from the other side of the room, who will learn the simpler exercises and is prepared to be instructed in the best method of carrying out the most fundamental tasks the handicapped child should perform, is the best friend of the child and the therapist.

Parents should be excluded from the treatment session when they interfere all the time or if they refuse to participate in the regime. Fortunately most parents are very willing to learn and eager to help.

With the slightly older child in the 4 to 8 years age group there can be vast differences in the mental capacity and approach. Children up to about the age of 5 will play on their own in a group environment and over the age of 5 will increasingly be willing to play with a partner. This development will increase the variety of exercises which can be used.

Children of this group will have developed interests and normal play patterns and enquiries should be made of the parents or the child observed in an assessment environment to allow suitable exercises to be chosen. The exercises should be briefly explained, but it will be necessary for the therapist to join in the activity and teach by example and thus by demonstration. Some enjoy a challenge and others need cajoling or encouragement and sometimes a great deal of shyness has to be overcome. Whatever the emotional approach the child should have a routine of exercises which is progressed regularly (and recorded). If no progress is being made the exercises should be altered if not progressed so that they do not seem to be in a rut. All children tend to have plateaux of performance in the same way that they have intermittent spurts of growing. Plateauing may be the explanation of lack of progress and approaching the exercise in another way may provide the required stimulus.

It is important to avoid the hazard of 'talking down' to children. A normal voice and manner of address appeals more to children who are charmed to be talked to in an adult voice and manner. A special vocabulary is not necessary, only remember that children have a limited vocabulary and known language. Failure to understand what is said will cause the child to say 'I don't know what you mean' or to fail to carry out the task. Then the explanation can be simplified.

An authoritative manner is also part of the therapist's role. Firm physical handling of a baby, firm commands to older children are necessary as the children must do their exercises. The same sort of command as to an adult, telling the child what to do, will give reassurance to a child who may, out of bewilderment, start to 'play up'.

Children from the age of 8 upwards are really small adults and apart from simplification of language to suit the age, can be dealt with as adults. It is important to remember that to many children imitative activities, e.g. role acting of being parents, nurses or at school is often not regarded as play. Play is, to some children, only going on when their own creative thoughts are being acted out with no relationship to the world of reality.

CHILDREN'S CLASSES (5–12 YEARS)

The best teachers are those who learn most from their pupils and there is no better material to learn from than children. They do not tolerate boredom and never hide their feelings. Young children are extremely vociferous, and whilst adults and older children may think the same, young children will actually tell you quite firmly 'I don't like you'. What they are telling you is that your method of communication does not please them. A therapist facing this situation would be well advised to investigate different methods or communication will eventually cease altogether. The following hints should be of help.

Most children coming to hospital for the first time are tense and frightened and a big effort must be made to provide a familiar atmosphere. Parents, who are emotionally tied up with their children, share this fear and the therapist should not take offence if this results in their abruptness and apparent lack of co-operation at the first treatment. As they see their child happily accepting the new situation they will become more cooperative.

It is a good idea if a special room can be set aside for the treatment of children. They tend to identify and associate deformed adults with grotesque characters in fairy tales and this only adds to their fears. The room should be reasonably small as children see things as being much bigger than they actually are and they tend to feel lost in a large open space. If a separate room is not possible, curtains could be used to divide a suitable area from a larger room. The room should be decorated with bright colours and one wall could be covered with pictures or posters, just like the classrooms at school. These will attract the child's attention and may well provide a topic of conversation between therapist and child, or between the new child and the other members of the class.

Overcoming the usual initial silence barrier in the very young is important. Children will chatter only when they feel secure and are therefore relaxed. In this atmosphere, they will be happy and cooperative. All children must have complete confidence in the therapist and she should have a little prior knowledge of each new child so that she can talk of familiar things and the child does not feel to be meeting a complete stranger. The therapist should make 'getting to know each other' her primary concern at the first treatment, and it is a help if a new child arrives a little before the rest of the class.

The therapist should take care not to tower over a child. It is a good idea to get down to his level by sitting or crouching adjacent to him and to greet him with a smile. She should try to encourage him to talk by asking questions about his family or pets so that he feels she is involved in his life away from hospital. The therapist must take care to remember all she is told and the child's trust in her will gradually grow, although a young child may need a few visits before he is completely at ease. Some young children respond to physical contact and a new child may like to perform his exercises while holding the therapist's hand. He will let go of his own accord when he becomes absorbed in the simple painfree exercises that should be taken at the beginning of the class.

At the first treatment the parent should be invited into the room and the therapist should tactfully ask her not to interrupt the class and assure her that there will be an opportunity for her to ask questions later. It should seldom be necessary for a parent to be excluded from a class. Sometimes the child requests this and, as the parent may later be criticizing the child's performance, the therapist should accede to the request until she can talk to the parent and assure herself that it will no longer happen. It is best to discuss problems whilst the child is otherwise gainfully occupied—perhaps when he is getting dressed as it is not a good thing to discuss the child when he is listening. If he thinks his physical difficulties are attracting his mother's attention at home it might slow down his progress, e.g. an asthmatic child may well bring on an attack in order to attract his mother's attention more to himself than to her other tasks. Each parent should be involved in the supervision of the exercises to be done at home, and this should make them feel useful. Parents should be advised how routine actions at home could help the child's progress, e.g. a child with flat feet should hang his coat on a peg high enough to make him lift on to his toes each time he takes it off and on.

In children's classes the age range should be small. The 5- to 8-year-old children will work well together, and children from 9 to 12 years old can be grouped together successfully. (Some 8-year-old children may be better in the older group.) Children in the younger group have a vivid imagination and will enjoy performing their exercises by acting out their own ideas of people and objects in a story told by the therapist. The children should be encouraged to add their own ideas to the story and the therapist should learn quickly to turn them into useful exercises. Many effective exercises for a chest class can be found in the story of a farmer riding on a tractor (the turning of wheels for shoulder mobilizing) to chop down trees and saw them into logs (trunk

rotation and side flexion). The logs then float down the river (relaxation) and are finally thrown on to a lorry (trunk flexion and extension). Imitation of wind blowing can produce deep breathing. It is essential that the story is told with great expression with the therapist involving herself in the movements.

Opportunity for working with a partner for some of the exercises is a good idea, but team work should be reserved for the older children. Young children will enjoy games where one child is the focal point, e.g. 'What time is it Mr Wolf' could be used to exercise feet. In the older age group the exercises should be taught in a more adult way and in both groups vocabulary and ideas used should be within their comprehension. The 9- to 12-year-old children particularly enjoy games involving teams.

There should be a variety of available apparatus, not all on show at once. It is a good idea if some of it is identifiable by the child as that used at home or at school. Apparatus makes the exercises more interesting and takes the child's attention from the part being exercised. Extra care should be taken in making sure the exercises are performed in safety. All children demand keen observation as they are impulsive and move quickly and suddenly without thought for their own or other's safety. The majority of exercises should allow freedom in standing positions unless the child's disability prevents this and then the starting positions used should be the most active possible. The concentration span of children is limited so that exercises should be of short duration and the therapist should prepare a greater variety and more exercises than she would for adult classes. Children are always enthusiastic and the therapist should make sure there are no long gaps between the exercises, as if this happens the children will find their own, often undesirable occupation, and control of the class will be quickly lost.

The therapist should give very brief explanations of exercises and be prepared to demonstrate and join in many of the activities. Children are always anxious to please and praise will lead to a big increase in effort. The therapist should look carefully for effort in those who find the exercises difficult and remember that praise is especially important to such children. Children like to be noticed, 'look at me' is a favourite phrase in the younger age group and the therapist should use this to encourage good and better work. All children like to demonstrate good work, but the therapist should take care that each child in turn is capable of demonstrating something or it could lead to unhappiness and a decrease in effort for a few. 'Follow my leader' type of exercises with different children playing the leader according to the difficulty of the exercise are good for encouraging all ranges of ability.

Clothing

The therapist's clothing should be colourful. It is unusual for mother or teacher to be dressed completely in white and the therapist is in a similar relationship with the children. Parents should be advised to bring young children in clothing that is suitable for exercise as they are often reluctant to undress, particularly in their early classes. It is best to suggest they remove clothing as the exercises make them hot, and they are therefore more readily persuaded to discard their clothes. The older age group will enjoy changing into a special outfit for exercises.

Lastly—though some children will appeal to the therapist more than others, evidence of favouritism will quickly lead to disaster.

CHAPTER 19

Special Regimes

M. HOLLIS

FRENKEL'S EXERCISES (SENSORY ATAXIA)

Patients who suffer total or partial sensory ataxia will lose both cutaneous and proprioceptive sensation and therefore tend to exaggerate movements in an attempt to complete them. Their disability is easily tested because patients with sensory loss perform a simple movement less smoothly and well with the eyes closed than with the eyes open. Their movements are also arhythmical and lack smoothness and precision.

The loss of proprioceptive impulses is compensated for by the use of vision and hearing. The movements must be performed accurately and with great precision and constant repetition of each movement is necessary until this is achieved. The patient must concentrate hard and watch the movement throughout while counting at a slow even tempo. No progression should be made until the first movement can be performed accurately. Adequate rest periods may be necessary during a treatment session as the patient may tire and lose the concentration necessary to achieve precision.

The rules are:

1 Every movement he performs must be watched by the patient and a high degree of concentration is required.
2 He must count out loud at first, then to himself at a slow even tempo and try to perform the same range of movement for each count with great precision.
3 The counting tempo must be the patient's own and not one imposed by the therapist.
4 Large single movements are retrained first, followed by alternate movements of contralateral limbs, then more complex movements.
5 Every movement made in the treatment session is counted at the same tempo and watched closely.
6 During performance the patient should be guarded against falls.
7 The worst limb should be exercised most.
8 Progression should not be made until smooth accurate performance of the first exercise is achieved and this rule is followed for all progressions.
9 Give the patient adequate periods of rest.

The regime starts when the order in which movements are to be trained has been decided. The patient is suitably positioned from both the point of view of maximum support to allow the part to be moved easily, and so that he can see the part moving through the selected range. The range of movement performed need not be the fullest possible range of the part, but should be that which can be easily managed and is functionally useful, e.g. in hip and knee flexion and extension—full extension is useful, flexion to 90° is all that is

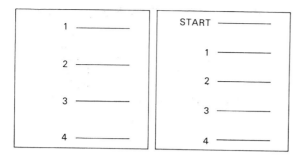

Figure 153 The marks for counting; A, to a count of 4; B, to a 'start' command and count of 4.

functionally necessary for sitting down in a chair.

A polished board or reasonably slippery surface is used. The two extremes of the selected range are decided upon and their positions on the supporting surface are marked with chalk. The distance between these two points is then marked out according to the agreed count. If the count is to include 'start, 1, 2, 3, 4' at which point the end of the range is reached then 5 marks are needed, but only 4 marks are required if the movement starts on the count of '1' (Figure 153).

The movement is first performed with the part supported. It is performed without pause during the movement first in one direction then in reverse and without wobbling. Next the patient can either lift the limb and touch each mark in turn or carry the limb through the air just off the support, passing each mark in turn.

Examples of movements are:

For the lower limb
   Side Lying—knee flexion and extension.
   Side Lying—hip flexion and extension.
   Half Lying—hip abduction and adduction.
   Half Lying—knee and hip flexion and extension.

For the upper limb
Sitting at a high table, arms held in abduction on the support
   Shoulder flexion and extension.
   Elbow flexion and extension.
   Elbow flexion with supination.
   Elbow extension with pronation.
   Wrist flexion and extension.

All the above exercises can then be practised:
1 With a voluntary halt.
2 With a halt on command.
3 With the part unsupported.
4 With the part unsupported and with a voluntary halt.
5 With the part unsupported and a halt on command.
6 Placing the heel or fingers on specific points.
7 As 6 with a voluntary halt, e.g. heel on opposite toes, ankle, shin and knee; fingers on opposite fingers, wrist, elbow and shoulder.
8 As 7 but halting on command.
9 As above but the therapist points to the part to be touched.
10 As above but the therapist moves her fingers as the patient reaches the part.

Next a less supported position can be used and the above stages used for each position and exercise such as:

   Sitting—knee extension and flexion.
   Sitting—hip abduction and adduction.
   Sitting—moving the foot over a numbered board or pushing a beanbag on the board (Figure 154).
   Sitting—lifting objects about on a table.
   Sitting—personal toilet training.

Walking training follows:

The patient stands using Stride Standing or

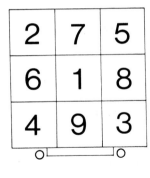

Chair legs

Figure 154 The numbered board for coordinated lower limb movements in sitting.

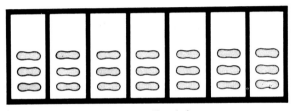

Figure 155 A Frenkel mat.

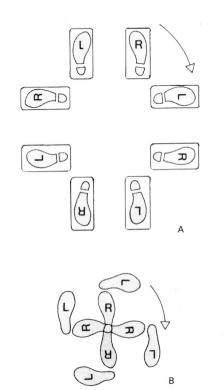

Figure 156 A, Step turning; B, Pivot turning. A is easier than B. When using B the patient will not necessarily be in line with his stepping line on the Frenkel mat.

Oblique Walk Standing while holding on a firm hand support (wall bars or fixed parallel bars). Weight transference is practised first remembering that counting must be maintained.

Sideways walking is practised first making the base narrower and wider in turn but never closing the base into Close Standing. A Frenkel mat can be used (Figure 155) when the patient is first required to put the foot into a space and eventually on to the lines.

Forward progression to ordinary walking with a wide base using first a 'step to' gait, i.e. right foot forwards, left foot up to it. Then later the left foot can be carried through and forwards. The two outer sets of footprints on the Frenkel mat are used first followed by using one of the outer and the middle footprints.

Turning round may be performed by either step turning or pivot and step turning.

Step turning The direction of the turn is decided upon, e.g. to the right. The right foot is lifted and turned through 90° and placed in the right-hand footprint. The left foot is lifted, turned and placed in the left-hand footprint (Figure 156,A). The above manoeuvres are continued until the patient has turned through 180° or 360°.

Pivot turning   A decision is again made about direction but this method may be used when the turn must be made in the direction of the worst leg. The patient pivots to the right on the heel of the right leg. The left foot is then lifted, turned and placed a short distance away alongside the first foot. The manoeuvre is repeated (Figure 156,B). Pivot turning may also be used as a progression on step turning as the base may be narrower.

VERTIGO

Vertigo occasionally requires a regime of exercises when it follows concussion as a post-concussion syndrome or when it is associated with space-occupying lesions or vascular accidents of the brain. It may also be used for conditions such as Ménière's disease which does not respond to drug therapy..

The regime of exercises is based on the principle of gradually inducing an attack of vertigo and then, when the patient recovers, carrying on with the regime. In this way the threshold of onset of an attack is pushed back and the patient learns both to accommodate to and to cope with an attack.

The regime starts with the patient performing eye movements while fully supported and continues through lessening support until the body movements can be made fast enough to evade moving obstacles.

The positions used are:
Lying with minimal pillows for comfort.
Half Lying.
Sitting in a corner of a room (i.e. using two walls for moral support).
Sitting free in a space.
Kneel Sitting.

Standing—Stride or Walk and eventually walking.

The objective is achieved by the therapist using a small coloured ball which she moves about in front of the fully supported patient asking him to follow the movements with his eyes. Next the range of the movement is increased so that head movements must be performed to keep the ball in sight.

In Half Lying a return is made to eye movements only and then to head movements again.

In Sitting the same procedure is followed. The ball can be bounced by the therapist then by the patient starting with a single bounce and catch, continuing with repetitive bouncing with either hand and in different areas round the patient. Throwing between patient and therapist follows with the therapist aiming the ball to make the patient move both or either arm to catch. In other words obtaining spontaneous displacement from the sitting and supported position and recovery to that position. Kneel Sitting is a position of security in which total body displacement can take place as the patient is required to retrieve objects placed further and further away.

Similar procedures to the above can be practised in free Sitting plus getting up from the stool and walking round it, first without, then with ball bouncing or throwing it in the air and catching.

An obstacle course is then set up and the patient is required to thread his way in and out of the course, to walk in tight circles round some of the obstacles at first carefully escorted by the therapist and then to cover the course with other people simultaneously using it from other directions. Such a course may be set up first indoors and then outdoors, or alternatively the patient should be taken on a walk in the grounds of the hospital and through the adjacent streets.

This regime can be taught to a group of patients once they are all able to sit on a chair or stool.

POSTURE

Posture is an alternative name for position but in an exercise context is usually taken to be a dynamic position in which the body components relate to one another so that the centre of gravity is over the base and the muscle work to maintain the position is reduced to a minimum.

Good posture is also pleasing to the eye and is dynamically adapted to the size of the base and the circumstances in which the body is resting or working. Good posture should not throw undue stress on muscle or joints and should be automatically resumed after displacement has occurred.

Poor posture is frequently produced by bad habits, e.g. the slouching posture adopted by the adolescent following the fashion of walking and standing with their hands in the front pockets of jeans. The use of unsuitable equipment may induce poor posture, e.g. a too low working surface will cause a kyphotic posture of the back at its weakest point; and associated round shoulders and poking chin will follow.

Holding the head to one side in a 'listening' posture due to slight deafness may become a bad habit and lead to the adoption of resultant deviations of the relationships of pelvis to shoulder girdle or of the vertebrae to one another.

Standing with most of the weight on one leg will lead to lateral deviations of the vertebrae and pelvis–shoulder girdle relationship. When the cause is shortness of the lower limb of more than 2·5 cm, correction will occur if raised footwear is worn but if any of the above postural habits are allowed to persist they will become permanent disfigurements and adaptive shortening of the soft tissues will ensue.

Early detection of poor posture and retraining to good position can be most rewarding and may need the following procedures.

a The patient's interest must be gained and he must *want* to improve his posture.
b Local relaxation may need to be taught, preferably in Lying.
c The patient is then 'straightened' by teaching the correct alignment of each body component to the other starting with the pelvis–shoulder girdle relationship. At this point the patient may complain that 'It, or he, feels odd'. The new proprioceptive pathways are being stimulated and he will now have to learn that 'feeling odd' may be correct. During this part of the proceedings he should be encouraged to maintain maximum body length by feeling as though he was stretching like a piece of elastic between his feet and his head.
d It is now important to displace body components while maintaining the corrected position, e.g. perform an arm or leg exercise and MAINTAIN the new posture.
e Next he must be totally displaced into a vigorous activity or maybe a game and then he must lie down and REGAIN his new posture.

This procedure can be repeated several times perhaps during the course of a class but at the first treatment the patient must also experience his corrected posture in Sitting and Standing and by constant reminder in all dynamic positions assumed during the course of that day's treatment session.

The treatment must include, for each patient, the adoption of their normal work or daily activity position so that the therapist can teach correction of what may be a poor posture adopted for the greater part of the day.

CHAPTER 20
A Neurophysiological View of Movement

P. J. WADDINGTON

The principles underlying the techniques used in movement form two major complementary sections, i.e. mechanical and physiological. Those which are called neurophysiological techniques stress this aspect while acknowledging the importance of and taking into account the mechanical principles. The terms central excitatory state and central inhibitory state may be used to describe the prolonged effects of excitatory or inhibitory influences upon the spinal cord.

'In view of the multiple, shifting and often antagonistic influences which constantly bombard the final common paths, it is surprising that chaos does not result.' William F. Ganong.

However, it is obvious that the normal individual is a highly coordinated, purposefully functioning organism. When taking the neurophysiological view of movement which is made abnormal through injury or disease, the therapist will have to consider how she wishes to influence the central nervous system to facilitate normal movement.

There are several neurophysiological methods, for example, Proprioceptive Neuromuscular Facilitation Techniques (P.N.F.), Bobath, Rood, Peto and Temple Fay; each one was developed independently in response to the many-sided problems of poor or abnormal movement. Each emphasizes a different aspect of the neurophysiological approach.

This section does not set out to teach these techniques but to give the student some insight into the basic concepts of the neurophysiological approach to movement. P.N.F. is explained in detail because of its value as a technique and as an introduction to normal patterns of movement. It also lays stress on the importance of accurate sensory input.

The neurodevelopmental approach of Karel and Berta Bobath also stresses the 'two way' aspect of sensory input; i.e. 'handling', the sensory input received by the patient from the therapist or parent and the sensory feedback of the individual's own movement whether it be normal or abnormal. This view has highlighted and influenced the approach taken here to tone, pattern and the less voluntary aspects of movement, particularly in the field of balance.

Thus there are two concepts to consider when selecting a technique.

1 The sensory-motor nature of movement.
2 The importance of tone. Movement occurs as a result of a coordinated change or adjustment of tone.

These two factors are interrelated.

Without sensory receptors and the constant bombardment of the nervous system with sensory information, only a small fraction of which reaches the level of consciousness, the individual would be unaware, either consciously or subconsciously, of his body image. He would be unaware of his starting position when preparing to move and of the effectiveness or accuracy of any movement achieved. The infant with abnormal tone and reflexes is unable to go through the normal developmental sequences necessary for the emergence of the mature locomotor system. He will have an abnormal background of sensory movement patterns because he has never moved normally. The adult patient may develop abnormal patterns as a result of a central nervous system lesion or following injury to the musculoskeletal system. Once established, an abnormal movement pattern is difficult to eradicate.

Abnormalities occur in muscle tone as a result of damage to the nervous system affecting the lower motor neurone, the upper motor neurone and/or the extrapyramidal system. Disease or injury affecting the lower motor neurone results in flaccidity of muscle. The muscle may be either totally paralysed or show a degree of weakness dependent upon the number of motor units involved. Lesions within the central nervous system may lead to a disturbance of the balance between excitatory and inhibitory influences on the motor neurone pools. Reduction in excitatory influences results in hypotonia, when the muscles are less sensitive to stretch. Hypertonia results from reduced inhibition and the response to stretch is abnormally high. There are two types of hypertonia, spasticity and rigidity.

Spasticity has been described as: 'That which is caused by a lesion in the corticospinal system resulting in hypertonicity, and a poor quality of voluntary movement. This latter being limited to a few or one only primitive, mass movement or pathological, mass movement patterns'. An example of spasticity may be seen in the classical hemiplegic patient.

Rigidity is an increase in tone which is equal in all muscle groups and maintained through the full range of movement, a pathological co-contraction, as seen in patients with Parkinson's disease. In normal individuals co-contraction, i.e. simultaneous contraction of agonists and antagonists making the limb into a rigid pillar, is exhibited in the positive supporting reaction and also during voluntary movements in the action of fixators and synergists.

Muscle tone may be raised in the normal individual following injury, this is called spasm. It is a normal protective mechanism resulting in limitation of movement.

For normal movement to occur, it is necessary for the individual to have normal tone. Movement is the result of coordinated muscle activity requiring the interaction of agonists, antagonists, synergists, and fixators. This coordinated activity results in a movement pattern. Although the normal adult is capable of numerous combinations of movements there is a basic framework which is recognized as forming *the normal adult patterns of movement*. Normal patterns are diagonal movements with a rotary component, they are used in such basic activities as rolling over, walking, kicking a ball, taking the hand to the mouth and writing.

These normal patterns are disturbed as a result of injury or disease of the locomotor system. Movements or postural patterns imposed on an individual as a result may be called *pathological patterns*, e.g. the hemiplegic adult, the spastic quadriplegic child and the patient with the painful arthritic hip are all instantly recognizable to the trained observer.

The patterns of movement of the infant,

frequently reflex in nature, may be called *primitive patterns.* These may be either normal or pathological. There are two deciding factors. The ability of a child to move and change its position and the pattern of movement related to the child's age, e.g.

1 Many infants may be seen to take up the position determined by the asymmetrical tonic neck reflex (A.T.N.R.), the vital difference being that the normal infant can move from the position, the spastic child is more or less fixed there.

2 Patterns of movement must always be compared with the child's age. The child at about 12 months old begins to walk, at first with a wide base using the upper limbs to aid balance. As balance begins to improve the child adopts the adult gait pattern, rotating the trunk and swinging the arms. The gait pattern which would be normal for the child at 12 months would be abnormal or pathological for an older child. It must be remembered that the developmental sequence is all important and that there is some latitude in the actual age at which certain activities and reflexes appear and disappear. Even the developmental sequence is not rigid, e.g. some children never crawl. As with all movement, experience in observing and handling is important for accurate assessment.

Thus, patterns of movement may be either normal or pathological and the basis for these patterns is tone.

How much movement is directly under willed voluntary control? Some activities such as tying shoe laces, fastening buttons and driving a car have to be painstakingly learnt as a direct effort of will, but once learnt these movements become more automatic and only impinge on the conscious mind if the sequence is disturbed, i.e. when sensory receptors alert

us, e.g. when the act of changing gear goes wrong. Standing and walking are less voluntary and are based on postural reflexes. If the individual's balance is disturbed, the activities necessary to restore balance are activated reflexly at subconscious level. Only when balance is seriously disturbed are we consciously aware of it and only then when it is too late to do anything about it.

If balance reactions fail, the protective extensor response or saving reaction is reflexly activated.

The protective withdrawal reflex, e.g. when touching an electric hotplate, occurs at spinal level, with the conscious reception of sensory information following a fraction of a second later. Even this is not as simple as it might seem, the withdrawal reflex is a pattern of total flexion, but to release something hot means that the hand must open; when the object is valuable, control may be exercised until it can be put down safely.

When considering any re-education programme, voluntary and involuntary aspects of movement have to be considered especially when retraining gait and balance. Movement has been likened to the iceberg, the smaller portion above the water is compared to the more voluntary movements and the larger submerged portion to the less voluntary activities.

The word facilitation means to make easy. Normal movement will be facilitated by bombarding the nervous system with as much helpful sensory information as possible. As a prelude it may be necessary to attempt to correct abnormalities of tone.

When the patient has muscle weakness uncomplicated by abnormal tone, he will require a programme of progressive resistance exercises. The advantage of using manual rather than other forms of resistance is that the therapist herself will learn to respond to the sensory input she receives from the patient. She will be able to adapt her grip to give the patient exactly the right sensory stimuli and throughout the movement she will be able to adjust the amount of resistance she gives.

The responsiveness of the therapist in handling the patient is a vital part of neurophysiological techniques whether she is dealing with voluntary or less voluntary movements. It is also essential in assessing and influencing muscle tone.

CHAPTER 21
Proprioceptive Neuromuscular Facilitation (P.N.F.)

P. J. WADDINGTON

This technique was developed by Herman Kabat, his work has been continued and expanded by Margaret Knott. Herman Kabat was interested in the treatment of 'patients with paralysis' and he stressed the importance of central excitation. The strength of a muscle contraction is directly proportional to the number of activated motor units, which obey the 'all or none' law. The functioning of these is dependent upon the degree of excitation of the motor neurones. Thus the basic aim of the method is to stimulate the maximum number of motor units into activity and to hypertrophy all the remaining muscle fibres.

The basic technique

The importance of the proprioceptors, in particular the muscle spindles, was recognized as a key factor in facilitating the contraction of muscles. It was also recognized that to hypertrophy and increase the power of muscles it is necessary to make them work maximally in accordance with the basic principles of progressive resistance exercises.

Stretch

The patterns of movement associated with this technique were evolved from the basic idea of stretching (not overstretching) muscles to stimulate the activity of the muscle spindles, i.e. the patterns evolved from the concept of stretch. The position of stretch, the lengthened position of the muscles, is the starting position of each pattern and this *stretch stimulus* is maintained throughout the movement. An additional advantage of the position of stretch is that any contraction of a muscle on stretch will result in movement and not just in 'taking up' the slack. A simple analogy is that when a child pulls the string to which his toy duck is attached, the duck will not move until the string is taut. This follows Beevor's axiom: 'The brain knows not of muscles but of movement'. This axiom supports the basic idea of working in functional, mass movement patterns rather than trying to activate individual muscles.

Later this concept was extended to the *stretch reflex* which is obtained by an additional stretch superimposed on the muscles in the stretch stimulus position usually at the outer range of the pattern. All the components of a pattern, particularly the rotary component, must be stretched simultaneously. It must be stressed that it is not excessive additional force, applied by the therapist, which elicits a stretch reflex but the skill with which she applies the stretch to the whole pattern. The reflex contraction of muscles and the movement brought about in this way can be used to initiate voluntary movement. The patient is instructed to make his effort to move to

174

coincide with the reflex movement brought about by the therapist. The stretch reflex can also be used to aid the response of a weak muscle and to establish rhythmic contractions. A stretch reflex may also be used to obtain a lengthening reaction of hypertonic muscles:

a By stimulating a contraction of the opposing muscle group, the hypertonic muscles (the antagonists) will reciprocally lengthen.

b By reflexly stimulating a contraction of the hypertonic group. This contraction will be followed by a relaxation phase or lengthening reaction of the same muscle group (c.f. the muscle twitch).

Patterns of movement

These are movements in a straight line, in a diagonal direction with a rotary component acting as the holding or stabilizing group, i.e. each pattern has three dimensions. For the patterns of the arms and legs these are flexion or extension, abduction or adduction and rotation (Figure 157). These diagonal movements also apply to the head and trunk.

The exact position of the diagonal is critical because muscles are stronger in pattern (in the groove) than out of pattern and the whole basis of the technique is to facilitate the contraction of muscles. The diagonal is in line with the oblique trunk muscles, e.g. the arm

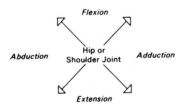

Figure 157 Diagram showing basic movement diagonals.

must only be an arm's width from the ear in the flexion, abduction and lateral rotation position, if the eyes and head are turned towards the hand in that position this will place the head and neck in the extension pattern with rotation to that side.

Patterns are named according to the direction of movement and therefore the finishing, not the starting, position. In completing the pattern the muscle contracts through full range from its lengthened to its shortened position.

Timing

The timing of the coordinated sequence of movements which form a pattern can be varied. In *normal timing* rotation initiates the movement, giving stability and direction to the pattern. Following this, movement will take place at the distal pivots (joints), e.g. fingers and wrist, and then at the proximal pivots, e.g. shoulder. Movement at the distal pivots must be completed before movement at the proximal pivots is completed. Changes in normal timing can be made to emphasize the contraction of a particular muscle group, i.e. *timing for emphasis*. This will be discussed later.

The grip

The therapist's grip is the key to facilitation. It provides four vital features.

1 Stretch—the correct grip enables the therapist to stretch all the components of a pattern simultaneously.

2 Exteroception—the grip must be such that it gives sensory stimulation to the skin in the direction of movement, i.e. the therapist's hands must not be on two surfaces at once.

3 Resistance—the grip must be such that the therapist is able to exert maximum resistance throughout the full range of movement.

4 Traction or approximation—the grip must be such that the therapist is able to exert either traction or approximation to the part as and when indicated.

This grip has been called by the author the '*lumbrical grip*' because it is essential for the therapist's hand on the patient's hand or foot to be flexed at the metacarpophalangeal joints and extended, but not rigidly so, at the interphalangeal joints. The more skilled the operator becomes the more selective and critical she is of her grip in the light of the patient's response.

Maximal resistance

The amount of resistance given by the therapist must be enough to demand from the patient his maximum effort. If the patient cannot lift the limb against gravity it will be necessary for the therapist to assist the movement. P.N.F. can be used to exercise muscles the strength of which relates to any point on the Oxford Classification (Chapter 12).

As with progressive resistance exercises using either weights or springs the therapist decides on the relationship between the number of repetitions and the amount of resistance. She may decide that the patient needs to repeat the movement many times, in which case the resistance will be reduced accordingly; conversely, the number of repetitions can be reduced and the resistance increased proportionately. The speed of the movement may also be controlled by varying the resistance.

The achievement and assessment of maximal resistance is related to the type of muscle work. For an *isotonic muscle contraction* the guide to maximal resistance is that the patient is able to perform a smooth, steady movement through full range; thus the amount of resistance may vary through different parts of the range.

For an *isometric muscle contraction*, where the rotary component (the holding or stabilizing group) is the dominant component, maximal resistance is developed slowly, i.e. the therapist gradually increases the resistance until the patient is making his maximum effort, taking care never to break the patient's hold.

Irradiation/overflow

Maximal resistance may be used to cause irradiation or overflow from stronger patterns to weaker patterns, or from stronger groups of muscles within a pattern to a weaker group within the same pattern (Chapter 25). This phenomenon is familiar to all therapists when strong, resisted dorsiflexion of the ankle is used to facilitate a contraction of the quadriceps. These two groups of muscles work functionally together in the walking pattern of the forward moving leg, i.e. flexion, adduction, with lateral rotation of the hip, extension of the knee and dorsiflexion of the ankle. No part of the body moves independently of other parts of the body. This reinforcement of activity in one area by activity elsewhere is the basis for the use of the overflow principle. Another example of reinforcement frequently used is to obtain a contraction of the abdominal muscles by flexing the neck against resistance, the resistance in most cases is provided by gravity, as the patient is positioned in Lying. If the neck flexors are strong and are made to work against maximal resistance the abdominal muscles will contract more strongly. Irradiation only occurs from strong muscles to weaker ones. Therefore, when planning a P.N.F. programme the therapist always starts with the patient's strongest patterns. The concept of reinforcement utilizes many of the primitive mass flexion and extension reflexes and the postural and righting reflexes.

When patients have spasticity, problems arise with the use of the irradiation principle, which requires the patient's maximal voluntary effort. When patients with spasticity are asked to work against maximal resistance *associated reactions* may occur. These appear to be movements but are in fact changes of tone and posture due to abnormalities in the central nervous system, i.e. they are pathological and should not be elicited. In individuals with normal tone *associated movements* occur, e.g. swinging the arms when walking, or gritting the teeth when making a great effort to unscrew a jar. These are normal activities and form part of the integrated action of the body.

It could be argued following the definition of maximal resistance for an isotonic muscle contraction, that when associated reactions occur, i.e. abnormal movements, the therapist is applying too much resistance.

The correct use of the concept of maximal resistance requires great skill and accurate assessment and observation.

Voice

To add to the total sensory input the therapist uses her voice to stimulate the patient's voluntary effort. The words of command are also vital in synchronizing the patient's voluntary effort with the stretch administered by the therapist. The action is preceded by the word '*now*' and this is followed by the command '*pull*' or '*push*'.

Joint structures

The proprioceptors in the joints are stimulated by the traction (a force tending to separate joint surfaces) or the approximation (a force tending to compress joint surfaces) applied by the therapist during the movement pattern. Traction is applied when the movement is occurring against gravity and approximation when the movement is occurring in the direction of the gravitational pull. Approximation may be used to activate postural reflexes.

Eyes

The patient is encouraged, when possible, to follow the movement with his eyes.

Thus, by summation of sensory input, the patient's natural movement patterns are facilitated; maximal resistance is used to strengthen muscles and the therapist's skills are augmented by the patient's maximum voluntary effort.

In the next section the basic normal patterns of movement, using normal timing, will be described, together with the therapist's stance and grip. It must be noted that the patterns alone do not constitute P.N.F. The basic principles must be applied to the patterns and then used in conjunction with additional techniques which may be classified as being either strengthening or relaxation techniques (obtaining a lengthening reaction of antagonists which are preventing movement into the agonist pattern). These techniques will be described in Chapter 25.

CHAPTER 22
P.N.F.
Arm Patterns

P. J. WADDINGTON

It is obvious that, to apply this method of treatment, the therapist must know the patterns and techniques in detail, but it is less obvious that the basis for success is the positioning and stance of the therapist; her balance, the use of her body weight and, as stressed before, the grip. For the patient to move in a diagonal direction smoothly against resistance, the therapist must be able to move smoothly herself using her body weight and not just her upper limbs when applying resistance.

The basic position for the therapist to take up is Lunge, with the forward foot pointing in the line of the movement diagonal and with the forward knee bent to give flexibility. The

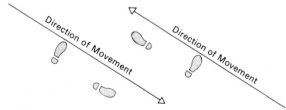

Figure 158 Diagram showing basic foot position in relationship to the movement diagonal.

rear foot is placed at right angles to the front foot to give stability (Figure 158).

The therapist must be positioned so that she can use her body weight to apply resistance and traction or approximation throughout the whole movement. She should be close enough to the part being exercised so that her back remains straight to ensure that the weight taken through her arms when applying resistance to gravity-assisted movements is transmitted to the floor without strain. All manually resisted exercise requires effort, but the work can be reduced and the dangers of strain can become negligible if the correct techniques are carefully learned and applied.

Grips and positions are described for the patient's right side. In the photographs which accompany each pattern, note the therapist's position. The patient should be positioned near to the side of the plinth to enable the therapist to obtain stretch on the flexion/ adduction patterns by taking the limb over the side of the plinth and to ensure that she is well balanced and does not overreach.

ARM PATTERNS

In P.N.F. terminology the term elevation is not used when referring to movements of the arm. Patterns in which the arm is raised above the head are called flexion patterns. Patterns are named according to the direction of

movement, i.e. the finishing position. There are two diagonals of movement in line with the oblique trunk muscles and four basic arm patterns (Figure 159).

In the basic arm patterns the elbow remains

178

straight throughout. However, each basic arm pattern may be adapted so that either elbow flexion or elbow extension takes place, for example:

Flexion/abduction/lateral rotation.
Flexion/abduction/lateral rotation with elbow flexion.
Flexion/abduction/lateral rotation with elbow extension.

Thus there are in effect twelve arm patterns, based on movements of the glenohumeral joint. It is obvious that movements of the shoulder girdle will accompany those of the upper limb. The movement patterns of the scapula will be described later (Chapter 24).

It is usual for the patient to be Supine although the patterns for the upper limb may be performed with the patient in Sitting.

When learning these patterns the patient may be taken through the movement passively. When resistance, i.e. maximal resistance, is applied the therapist must be guided as to the amount of resistance she gives by the fact that the patient always remains in the 'groove', i.e. does not deviate from the pattern. Once the movement has been learned resistance may be increased.

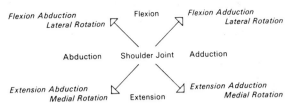

Figure 159 Diagram showing the shoulder movement in the four basic arm patterns.

Flexion/abduction/lateral rotation

Starting position (Figure 160)

PATIENT Extension/adduction/medial rotation of the shoulder with pronation of the forearm, flexion and ulnar deviation of the wrist, flexion of the fingers and flexion and opposition of the thumb.

THERAPIST
Stance The therapist stands in Lunge looking towards the patient's feet with her weight on the forward right leg and parallel with the proposed line of movement at the level of the patient's upper arm. During the movement the therapist transfers her weight from the forward right foot to the left foot and rotates so that she can watch the patient's hand throughout the movement.
Grip The therapist grasps the patient's right hand with her left (Figure 161). Note that because of the flexion of the metacarpo-

phalangeal joints only her fingers, thumb and thenar eminance are in contact with the dorsum of the patient's hand.

Commands

The therapist prepares the patient with the word '*now*', applies stretch to establish the stretch stimulus and gives the executive word '*push*'. After the movement has started, the therapist places the fingers of her right hand on the extensor surface of the patient's wrist approaching from the radial side (Figure 162). If the wrist and finger movements are slow to develop, extra resistance given by the hand on the wrist will facilitate these movements.

Movement

Extension of the fingers (particularly middle

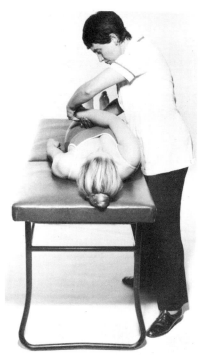

Figure 160 Starting position for the flexion/abduction/lateral rotation pattern of the arm.

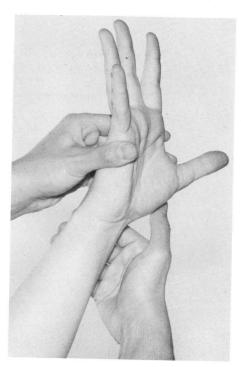

Figure 162 Grip—part way through the flexion/abduction/lateral rotation pattern of the arm.

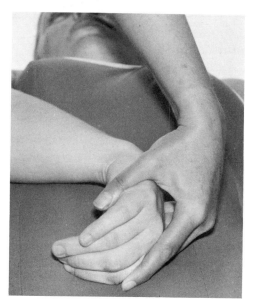

Figure 161 Grip—starting position for the flexion/abduction/lateral rotation pattern of the arm.

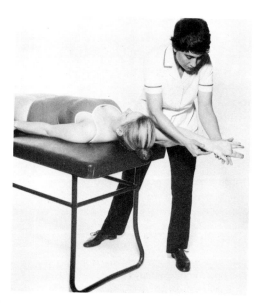

Figure 163 Finishing position for the flexion/abduction/lateral rotation pattern of the arm.

and index) and thumb, extension of the wrist with radial deviation, supination of the forearm, flexion, abduction and lateral rotation at the glenohumeral joint, rotation, elevation and adduction (retraction) of the scapula.

In normal timing, movement is initiated by the rotary component. Movement then occurs at the distal joints, to be followed in succession by the more proximal joints. Rotation continues throughout the pattern.

When the pattern is completed the arm should be about an arm's width from the patient's ear (Figure 163).

Flexion/abduction/lateral rotation with elbow flexion

Starting position

PATIENT   As for the basic pattern.
THERAPIST   *Stance* and *grip* as for the basic pattern except that the therapist's right hand is placed over the lateral epicondyle of the humerus to encourage flexion. She may also slip her thumb into the elbow crease.

Movement

As for the basic pattern with the addition of elbow flexion (Figure 164).

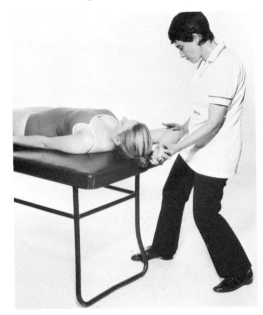

Figure 164   Finishing position for the flexion/abduction/lateral rotation with elbow flexion pattern of the arm.

Flexion/abduction/lateral rotation with elbow extension

Starting position (Figure 165)

PATIENT   As for the basic pattern with the addition of elbow flexion.
THERAPIST
Stance   The therapist takes up Lunge position near to the patient's head.
Grip   She places her right hand over the lateral epicondyle and the point of the elbow to encourage extension, and with the left hand grips the patient's hand as for the basic pattern.

Movement

As for the basic pattern with the addition of elbow extension.

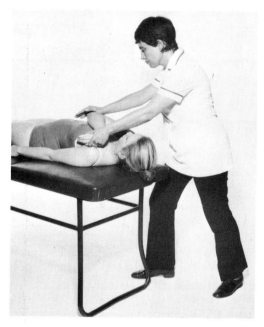

Figure 165 Starting position for the flexion/abduction/lateral rotation with elbow extension of the arm.

Extension/adduction/medial rotation

Starting position

PATIENT Flexion/abduction/lateral rotation with supination of the forearm, extension of the wrist with radial deviation and extension of the fingers and thumb.

THERAPIST

Stance The therapist's feet remain in the same place as for the antagonist pattern, i.e. flexion/abduction/lateral rotation, but the Lunge stance is reversed, the therapist faces the patient's outstretched hand with her left foot forwards and with the knee flexed. During the movement the therapist transfers her weight from the forward left foot to the right foot.

Grip The therapist places the palm of her right hand into the palm of the patient's right hand and grasps the palm with the lumbrical grip ensuring that the fingers do not flex and exert pressure on the dorsum of the patient's hand (Figure 166). The therapist places the fingers of her left hand on the flexor surface of the wrist approaching from the radial side. If the movement at the wrist is inadequate, additional resistance at the wrist will stimulate activity.

Commands

The therapist prepares the patient for movement with the word '*now*', applies stretch to establish the stretch stimulus and then instructs the patient to '*grip my hand and pull down*'.

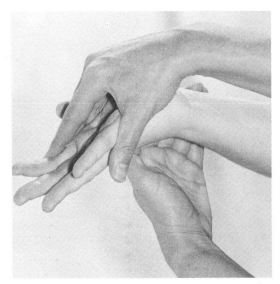

Figure 166 Grip—starting position for the extension/adduction/medial rotation pattern of the arm.

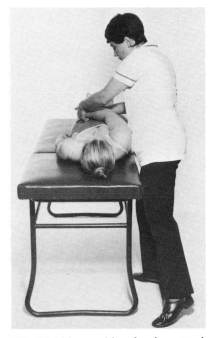

Figure 167 Finishing position for the extension/adduction/medial rotation pattern of the arm.

Movement

Flexion of the fingers (with particular emphasis on the index and middle fingers), opposition of the thumb, flexion of the wrist with ulnar deviation, pronation of the forearm, extension, adduction, medial rotation at the glenohumeral joint, depression, abduction of the scapula (Figure 167).

In normal timing movement is initiated by the rotary component. Movement then occurs at the distal joints to be followed in succession by the more proximal joints. Rotation continues throughout the pattern.

Extension/adduction/medial rotation with elbow flexion

Starting position

PATIENT   As for the basic pattern.

THERAPIST

Stance   The therapist moves her feet nearer to the patient's hand than for the straight arm pattern.

Grip   This is one of the rare occasions when the grip on the hand does not remain the same for the three similar patterns. The grip is changed so that at the end of the movement the therapist does not find her own arms crossed. The therapist places the palm of her left hand within the patient's outstretched right hand and the fingers of her right hand over the flexor aspect of the patient's elbow to encourage elbow flexion.

Movement

As for the basic pattern with the addition of elbow flexion. Care must be taken to ensure that the arm moves in the diagonal direction as it can easily complete the movement at the patient's side (Figure 168).

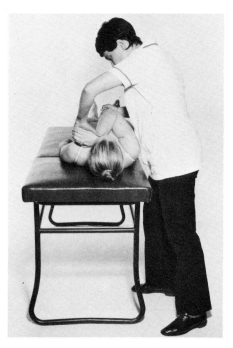

Figure 168 Finishing position for the extension/adduction/medial rotation with elbow flexion pattern of the arm.

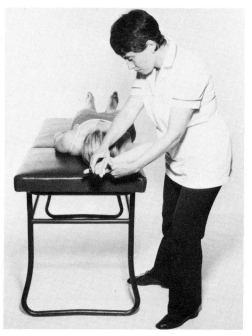

Figure 169 Starting position for the extension/adduction/medial rotation with elbow extension pattern of the arm.

Extension/adduction/medial rotation with elbow extension

Starting position (Figure 169).

PATIENT As for the basic pattern with the addition of elbow flexion.
THERAPIST *Stance* and *grip* as for the basic pattern.

In the *flexion/abduction–extension/adduction* diagonal the thumb and radial side of the limb lead throughout the movement. It is in this diagonal, in which opposition of the thumb

Movement

As for the basic pattern with the addition of elbow extension.

occurs, that many of the highly skilled movements take place, e.g. writing and threading a needle. The index and middle fingers also work to advantage.

Flexion/adduction/lateral rotation

Starting position (Figure 170)

PATIENT Extension/abduction/medial rotation of the shoulder with pronation of the forearm, extension with ulnar deviation of the wrist, extension of the fingers, extension and abduction of the thumb. The therapist must ensure that the patient is near enough to the side of the plinth to enable the arm to be taken into extension beyond the horizontal. The patient's arm should only be abducted to about an arm's width from the side of the body. It is possible to test for the correct position as muscles are stronger in pattern. Care must be taken to ensure that the patient's fingers are fully extended before the movement begins.

THERAPIST

Stance The therapist stands at the level of the patient's upper arm in the Lunge position facing the patient's feet and with her weight on her forward right foot and parallel with the proposed line of movement. During the movement the therapist transfers her weight from the right to the left foot rotating so that she can continue to watch the patient's hand throughout the movement.

Grip The therapist grasps the patient's right hand by placing her left palm into the patient's palm approaching from the radial side. She uses the lumbrical grip thus ensuring that she does not touch the extensor surface of the patient's hand. The fingers of her right hand are placed on the flexor surface of the patient's

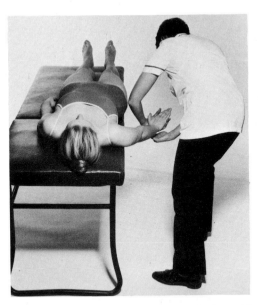

Figure 170 Starting position for the flexion/adduction/lateral rotation pattern of the arm. (In order to show the grip, the arm has been taken too far into abduction.)

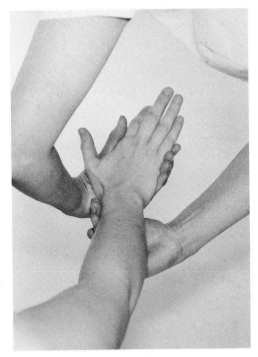

Figure 171 Detail of grip—starting position for the flexion/adduction/lateral rotation pattern of the arm.

wrist approaching from the ulnar side (Figure 171). The therapist may delay positioning her right hand until just after the movement has started.

Commands

The therapist prepares the patient for the movement by saying '*now*' and then follows this with the command '*grip my hand, pull up and across your nose*'.

Movement

Flexion of the fingers, particularly the little and ring fingers, adduction and flexion of the thumb, flexion of the wrist towards the radial side, supination of the forearm, flexion, adduction and lateral rotation at the gleno-humeral joint, rotation, elevation and abduction (protraction) of the scapula (Figure 172). As in all normal timing the movement is initiated by the rotary component. Movement then occurs at the distal joints to be followed in succession by the more proximal joints until the whole limb is moving.

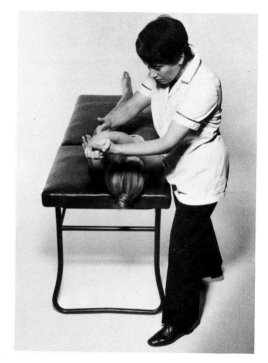

Figure 172 Finishing position for the flexion/adduction/lateral rotation pattern of the arm.

Flexion/adduction/lateral rotation with elbow flexion

Starting position

PATIENT   As for the basic pattern.
THERAPIST   *Stance* and *grip* as for the basic pattern. The therapist may move her right hand nearer to the patient's elbow.

Movement

As for the basic pattern with the addition of elbow flexion. This is the eating pattern. It may have been noted when practising the straight arm pattern that the patient has a tendency to want to flex at the elbow (Figure 173).

Flexion/adduction/lateral rotation with elbow extension

Starting position (Figure 174)

PATIENT   As for the basic pattern with the addition of elbow flexion.

THERAPIST   *Stance* and *grip* as for the basic pattern.

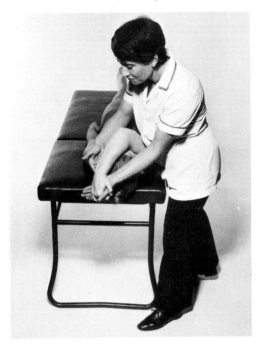

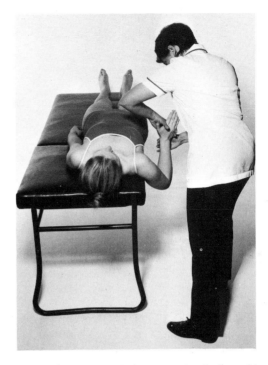

Figure 173 Finishing position for the flexion/adduction/lateral rotation with elbow flexion pattern of the arm.

Figure 174 Starting position for the flexion/adduction/lateral rotation with elbow extension pattern of the arm.

Movement

As for the basic pattern with the addition of elbow extension. Note this may seem a strange movement at first but a boxer has said that the pattern has the fundamental components of the 'upper cut'.

Extension/abduction/medial rotation

Starting position

PATIENT Flexion/adduction/lateral rotation, supination of the forearm, flexion and radial deviation of the wrist, flexion of the fingers and flexion and adduction of the thumb.

THERAPIST

Stance The therapist stands in the Lunge position facing the patient's head at the level of the patient's upper arm with her weight on her forward left foot and parallel with the proposed line of movement. During the movement the therapist transfers her weight from the left to the right foot, rotating so that she can continue to watch the patient's hand.

Grip The therapist, using her right hand and the lumbrical grip, grasps the dorsum of the patient's right hand ensuring that stretch is

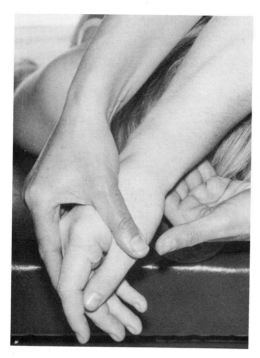

Figure 175 Grip—starting position for the extension/abduction/medial rotation pattern of the arm.

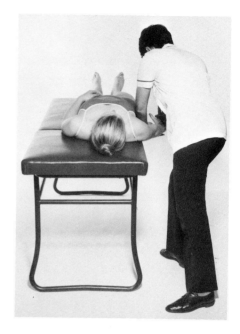

Figure 176 Finishing position for the extension/abduction/medial rotation pattern of the arm.

obtained and that emphasis is given by pressure with her fingers to the exteroceptors on the ulnar side of the patient's hand. After the movement has started the fingers of the therapist's left hand are placed on the extensor surface of the patient's wrist approaching from the flexor aspect and round the ulnar border, i.e. from between the patient's arm and body (Figure 175).

Commands

'*Now*'—'*push*'.

Movement

Extension of the fingers particularly the little and ring fingers, extension and abduction of the thumb, extension of the wrist towards the ulnar side, pronation of the forearm, extension, abduction and medial rotation of the gleno-humeral joint, rotation, depression and adduction of the scapula (Figure 176). As in all normal timing the movement is initiated by the rotary component, movement then occurs at the distal joints to be followed in succession by the more proximal joints until the whole limb is moving.

Extension/abduction/medial rotation with elbow flexion

Starting position

PATIENT As for the basic pattern.

THERAPIST *Stance* and *grip* of the right hand as for the basic pattern but the fingers of the left hand are placed over the point of the elbow approaching from the ulnar side to encourage elbow flexion.

Movement

As for the basic pattern with the addition of elbow flexion. This pattern can be seen in photographs of footballers kicking a ball, particularly when these photographs are 'posed' (Figure 177).

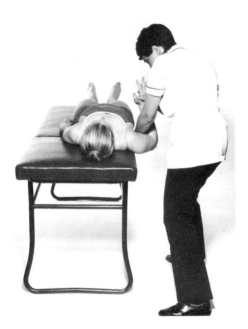

Figure 177 Finishing position for the extension/abduction/medial rotation with elbow flexion pattern of the arm.

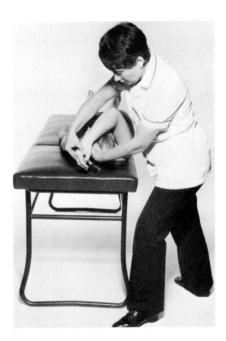

Figure 178 Starting position for the extension/abduction/medial rotation with elbow extension pattern of the arm.

Extension/abduction/medial rotation with elbow extension

Starting position (Figure 178)

PATIENT As for the basic pattern with the addition of elbow flexion.

THERAPIST *Stance* and *grip* as for the basic pattern.

Movement

As for the basic pattern with the addition of elbow extension. This movement occurs in eating when the hand is returning from the mouth.

In the *flexion/adduction–extension/abduction* diagonal the little finger and ulnar side of the limb lead throughout the movement. This is the diagonal of the eating pattern.

Thrust patterns

There are two additional patterns of the upper limb, the *thrust patterns*. One pattern has a flexion, the other an extension component. They are both adduction patterns with elbow extension, in which the rotation occurs in the opposite direction to the basic pattern and flexion of the wrist and fingers is replaced by extension. The addition of these two, to the basic twelve patterns, emphasizes the versatility of movement in the upper limb.

Thrust patterns are powerful movements. They can occur in any position; in Prone they are used to support the body on the hands as in 'press-ups'. The movement also occurs when reaching for an object with an opening hand in preparation for grasping.

Thrust into flexion/adduction

Starting position (Figure 179)

PATIENT Extension/abduction (an arm's width from the body) with lateral rotation of the shoulder, flexion of the elbow, supination of the forearm, wrist flexion with radial deviation and flexion of the fingers and thumb.

THERAPIST

Stance The therapist stands at the head of the plinth (as for manual cervical traction) with her right foot forwards in the Lunge position. *Grip* She places her left hand over the patient's right hand grasping the extensor surface giving pressure with her fingers on the ulnar side of the hand. Her right hand is placed with the thumb abducted over the flexor aspect of the upper arm and into the bend of the elbow. The author prefers this stance and grip but the therapist, if she chooses, may take up her stance as for the basic flexion/adduction/lateral rotation pattern.

Commands

'*Now*'—'*thrust*'. The use of the word thrust appears to have greater impact than push in this situation.

Movement

Protraction of the scapula, flexion, adduction

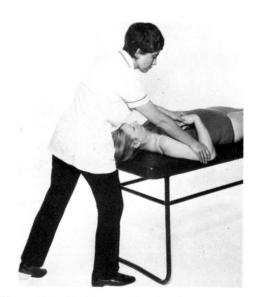

Figure 179 Starting position for the thrust pattern into flexion/adduction.

and medial rotation of the glenohumeral joint with elbow extension, wrist extension to the ulnar side, extension of the fingers and thumb (Figure 180). This pattern may be reversed in which case the therapist slips the fingers of her left hand into the patient's palm from the ulnar side and places her right hand on the point of the elbow.

Thrust into extension/adduction

Starting position

PATIENT Flexion/abduction/medial rotation of the shoulder, elbow flexion (so that the hand is on the shoulder), pronation of the forearm, wrist flexed towards the ulnar side, flexion of the fingers and thumb.

THERAPIST The therapist may stand in one of two positions each requiring a different grip.

1 *Stance* In Lunge position as for the basic extension/adduction pattern.

Grip The therapist places her left hand on the extensor surface of the patient's hand obtaining stretch by exerting pressure through her fingers. The therapist's right hand is placed on the upper arm (Figure 181,A).

2 *Stance* The therapist stands in the Lunge position with right foot forwards on the patient's left side (i.e. the opposite side to the arm being exercised) facing the patient's head.

Grip The therapist places her left hand over the extensor surface of the patient's hand obtaining stretch by exerting pressure on the radial side of the hand through her thumb. (This is one of the very few occasions when pressure is exerted through the thumb and not the fingers.) The therapist places her right

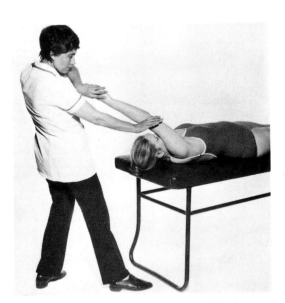

Figure 180 Finishing position for the thrust pattern into flexion/adduction.

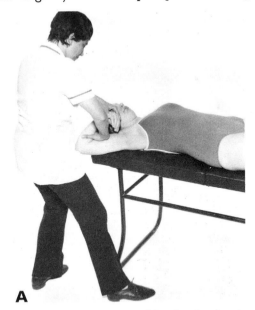

Figure 181 A, Starting position for the thrust pattern into extension/adduction.

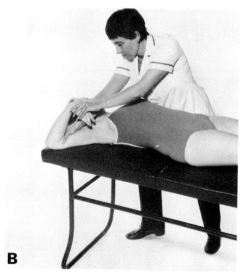

B

Figure 181   B, Alternative starting position for the thrust pattern into extension/adduction.

hand, thumb abducted and extended on the flexor surface of the patient's upper arm (Figure 181,B).

Commands

'*Now*'—'*thrust*'.

Movement

Protraction of the scapula, extension, adduction, lateral rotation of the glenohumeral joint, elbow extension, supination, wrist extension to the radial side, extension of the fingers and thumb (Figure 182A,B).

This pattern may be reversed. Reversals are more easily done if the therapist takes up starting position 2. The therapist slips the fingers of her left hand into the patient's palm from the ulnar side and places her right hand over the olecronan process.

Figure 182   B, Alternative finishing position for the thrust pattern into extension/adduction.

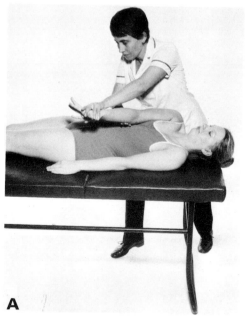

A

Figure 182   A, Finishing position for the thrust pattern into extension/adduction.

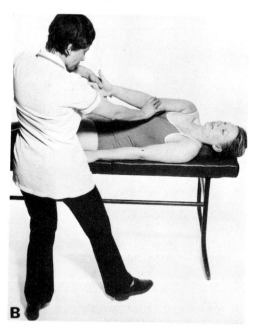

B

CHAPTER 23

P.N.F. Leg Patterns

P. J. WADDINGTON

As with the arm there are two diagonals of movement (Figure 183) in line with the

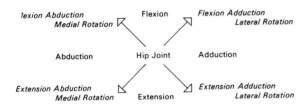

Flexion Abduction
Medial Rotation

Flexion

Flexion Adduction
Lateral Rotation

Abduction

Hip Joint

Adduction

Extension Abduction
Medial Rotation

Extension

Extension Adduction
Lateral Rotation

Figure 183 Diagram showing the hip movements in the four basic leg patterns.

oblique trunk muscles and four basic patterns.

In the basic leg patterns the knee remains straight throughout. However, each basic pattern may be adapted so that either knee flexion or knee extension takes place, for example:

flexion/adduction/lateral rotation
flexion/adduction/lateral rotation with knee flexion
flexion/adduction/lateral rotation with knee extension

Thus there are twelve leg patterns, based on the hip joint. It should be noted that throughout the movements the heel should lead the way.

It is usual for the patient to be Supine on a plinth.

Flexion/adduction/lateral rotation

Starting position (Figure 184)

PATIENT Extension/abduction/medial rotation of the hip, plantarflexion and eversion of the foot and flexion of the toes.

The patient lies at the side of the plinth so that the leg can be taken into full extension over the side without too much abduction which would take it out of pattern.

THERAPIST

Stance The therapist stands in the Lunge position in line with the diagonal of movement and with the forward left foot about level with the patient's foot. The therapist's weight is on the right foot so that her body weight can be used to exert traction. Both her knees are flexed.

Grip The therapist holds the patient's heel with her left hand and places her right hand over the dorsum of the patient's foot and uses the 'lumbrical grip'. With her thumb on the lateral border and fingers spread out on the medial border of the foot she exerts pressure through her fingers to give the correct exteroception and stretch (Figures 185, 186).

193

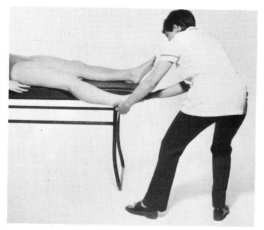

Figure 184 Starting position for the flexion/adduction/lateral rotation pattern of the leg.

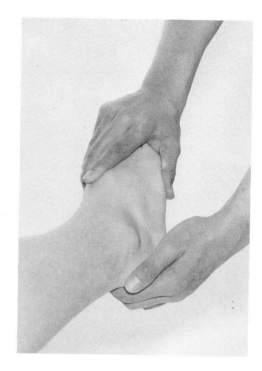

Figure 186 Grip (both hands)—starting position for the flexion/adduction/lateral rotation pattern of the leg.

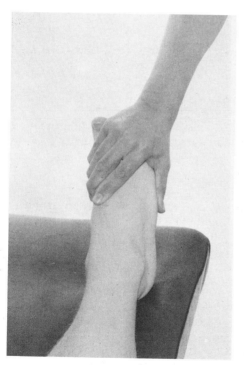

Figure 185 Basic grip for the hand placed on the patient's foot in the flexion/adduction/lateral rotation pattern of the leg.

Commands

'*Now*' used as a preparation for action. '*Turn your heel in and pull your foot up.*' The patient may respond initially and certainly will later to the simple commands '*now*'—'*pull*'.

Movement

In this pattern the therapist must pivot on her forward left foot taking a forward step with her right foot so that she is able to maintain her grip on the foot of the extended leg.

The position of the therapist's left hand also changes quickly. Once the rotation has started her left hand is placed on the extensor and adductor aspects of the patient's leg at the level of the knee. The patient's movement is lateral rotation of the hip, inversion and dorsiflexion of the foot and extension of the toes, followed by flexion and adduction at the hip (Figure 187).

In normal timing movement is initiated by the rotary component. Movement then occurs at the distal joints to be followed in succession by the more proximal joints. Rotation continues throughout the pattern. The length of the patient's hamstring muscles will determine the range of movement.

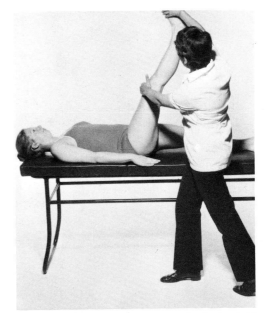

Figure 187 Finishing position for the flexion/adduction/lateral rotational pattern of the leg.

Flexion/adduction/lateral rotation with knee flexion

Starting position

PATIENT   As for flexion/adduction/lateral rotation.

THERAPIST
Stance   The therapist stands as for the flexion/adduction/lateral rotation pattern.
Grip   As for the flexion/adduction/lateral rotation pattern.

Commands

'*Now*'—'*pull up and bend your knee*'.

Movement

As the patient's knee flexes in this pattern it is not necessary for the therapist to take a step, it is sufficient for her to flex the forward left knee and perhaps glide forwards a little. The therapist's weight is transferred from the rear right foot to the forward left foot.

The patient's movement is as for the flexion, adduction, lateral rotation pattern with the addition of knee flexion. The therapist must ensure that knee flexion is active and resisted throughout the pattern by using her right hand, otherwise flexion can be brought about passively by gravity.

It is very easy to allow incorrect medial rotation to occur in this pattern if the knee is allowed to lead and the foot to follow in the movement diagonal. The therapist must ensure that the knee and foot move across diagonally together maintaining a vertical relationship to each other (Figure 188).

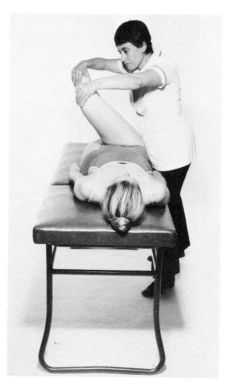

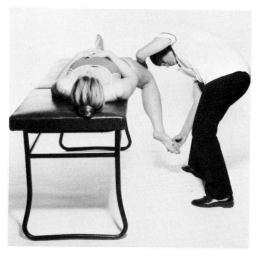

Figure 188 Finishing position for the flexion/adduction/lateral rotation with knee flexion pattern of the leg.

Figure 189 Starting position for the flexion/adduction/lateral rotation with knee extension pattern of the leg.

Flexion/adduction/lateral rotation with knee extension

Starting position (Figure 189)

PATIENT As for flexion/adduction/lateral rotation but with the knee flexed.

THERAPIST

Stance The therapist stands adjacent to the patient's flexed knee in the Lunge position facing the foot of the plinth, i.e. right foot forwards and knee flexed and her weight through the flexed left leg.

Grip The therapist grasps the foot with her right hand as before, slightly adapting her grasp to accommodate her changed stance.

She places her left hand on the extensor and adductor aspect of the patient's knee. Care must be taken not to overstretch rectus femoris in this position.

Commands

'*Now*'—'*turn your heel in and straighten your knee*'.

Movement

As before with the addition of knee extension.

To accommodate the adduction movement the therapist, having transferred her weight to the forward right foot, takes a step towards the plinth with her left foot.

Extension/abduction/medial rotation

Starting position

PATIENT　Flexion/adduction/lateral rotation of the hip, dorsiflexion and inversion of the foot, extension of the toes.

THERAPIST

Stance　The therapist faces the head of the plinth in Lunge in the line of the basic diagonal. She is near to the patient's hip and with the left foot forwards.

Grip　The therapist places her right hand held slightly in the 'lumbrical position' on the plantar surface of the patient's foot, with the thumb, in line with the palm, lying under the toes in a position to resist flexion. The therapist

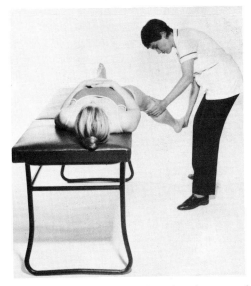

Figure 191　Finishing position for the extension/abduction/medial rotation pattern of the leg.

exerts pressure through her fingers on the medial border of the foot (Figure 190). The therapist stretches her left hand and places the thumb on the lateral surface of the patient's thigh near to the knee with the border of the index finger on the posterior aspect of the thigh. As the patient extends the leg this hand is in a position to catch and control the knee.

Commands

'*Now*'—'*turn your heel out and push your toes down*'. The patient may respond to the simple commands '*now*'—'*push*'.

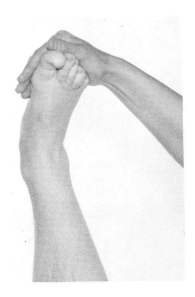

Figure 190　Grip on the foot—starting position for the extension/abduction/medial rotation pattern of the leg.

Movement

Medial rotation of the hip, plantarflexion and eversion of the foot, flexion of the toes and extension and abduction of the hip (Figure 191).

In normal timing movement is initiated by the rotary component. Movement then occurs at the distal joints to be followed in succession by the more proximal joints. Rotation continues throughout the pattern. The therapist transfers her weight from the left to the right foot and flexes her knee.

Extension/abduction/medial rotation with knee flexion

Starting position

PATIENT   As for extension/abduction/medial rotation.

THERAPIST   *Stance* and *grip* as for extension/abduction/medial rotation except that the left hand is placed slightly more proximally so that it will not impede knee flexion.

Commands

'*Now*'—'*turn your heel out, push your toes down and bend your knee*'.

Movement

Medial rotation of the hip, plantarflexion and eversion of the foot, flexion of the toes, knee flexion, extension and abduction of the hip. The therapist, having transferred her weight onto the forward right foot, takes a step to the side with her left foot to allow room for the patient's foot (Figure 192).

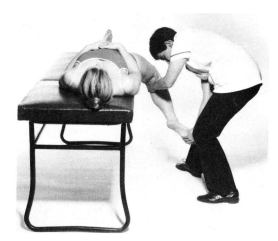

Figure 192 Finishing position for the extension/abduction/medial rotation with knee flexion pattern of the leg.

Extension/abduction/medial rotation with knee extension

Starting position (Figure 193)

PATIENT   Flexion/adduction/lateral rotation of the hip with knee flexion, dorsiflexion and inversion of the foot and extension of the toes. The therapist must ensure that the knee and foot are in the line parallel with the side of the plinth and the resting leg, i.e. that the hip is in lateral rotation. It is easy to deviate from this so that the knee and foot are diagonally related to each other. In this position the hip is medially rotated.

THERAPIST

Stance   The therapist stands facing the patient in Lunge position with her weight on the forward left leg.

Grip   As for the extension/abduction/medial rotation pattern.

Commands

'*Now*'—'*push*'.

Movement

Medial rotation of the hip, plantarflexion and eversion of the foot, flexion of the toes, extension of the knee and extension and abduction of the hip.

This pattern and the other mass extension pattern of the leg, i.e. extension/adduction/lateral rotation with knee extension are the strongest patterns in the body.

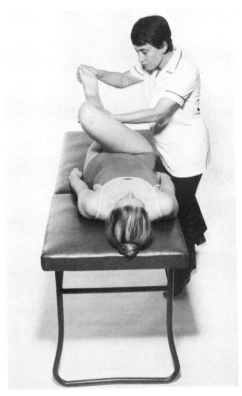

Figure 193 Starting position for the extension/abduction/medial rotation with knee extension pattern of the leg.

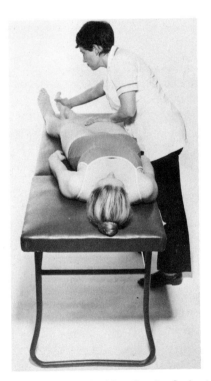

Figure 194 Starting position for the flexion/abduction/medial rotation pattern of the leg.

Flexion/abduction/medial rotation

Starting position (Figure 194)

PATIENT Extension/adduction/lateral rotation of the hip, plantarflexion and inversion of the foot and flexion of the toes.

To allow the leg to be adducted the other leg must be taken into abduction. In this

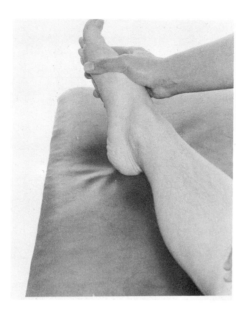

Figure 195 Grip on the foot—starting position for the flexion/abduction/medial rotation pattern of the leg.

position the final few degrees of extension cannot be obtained.

THERAPIST

Stance   The therapist stands in Lunge position at the level of the patient's thigh facing the foot of the plinth and with her right foot forwards.

Grip   The therapist places her right hand, using the lumbrical grip, on the dorsum of the patient's foot and, by exerting pressure through the fingers, she is able to obtain stretch (Figure 195). The left hand is placed on the upper and outer aspect of the thigh.

Commands

'*Now*'—'*turn your heel out and pull your foot up*'. This may later be reduced to '*now*'—'*pull up*'.

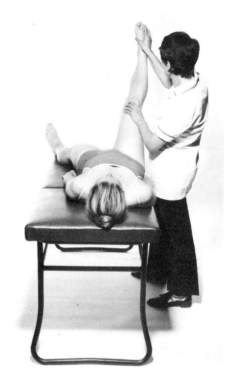

Figure 196 Approaching the finishing position for the flexion/abduction/medial rotation pattern of the leg.

Movement

Medial rotation of the hip, dorsiflexion and eversion of the foot, extension of the toes and flexion and abduction of the hip (Figure 196). In normal timing movement is initiated by the rotary component. Movement then occurs at the distal joints to be followed in succession by the more proximal joints. Rotation continues throughout the pattern.

To ensure good balance the therapist must transfer her weight to the rear left leg as the movement proceeds.

Flexion/abduction/medial rotation with knee flexion

Starting position

PATIENT   As for flexion/abduction/medial rotation.

THERAPIST
Either   *Stance* and *grip* as for flexion/abduction/medial rotation.
Or (Figure 197)
Stance   The therapist stands in the Lunge position, right foot forwards, facing the patient on the opposite side of the plinth, i.e. when the patient's right leg is being exercised she stands on the patient's left. The forward right foot is placed at about the level of the patient's right ankle and her weight is on the left foot. It is usual when using this method to cross the patient's active leg over the resting leg.

Grip   The therapist places her left hand on the dorsum of the patient's foot exerting pressure through her fingers. Her right hand may be placed under the patient's heel, pressure is given to the lateral aspect, otherwise it is placed on the lateral aspect of the thigh.

Commands

'*Now*'—'*pull*'.

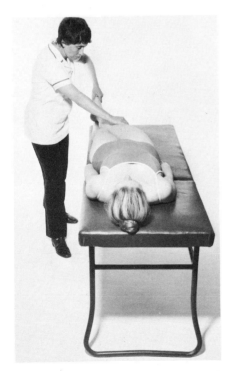

Figure 197   Alternative starting position for the flexion/abduction/medial rotation with knee flexion pattern of the leg.

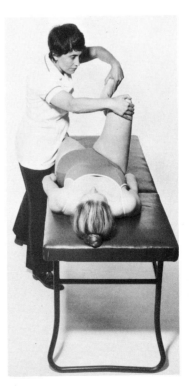

Figure 198   Approaching the finishing position for the flexion/abduction/medial rotation with knee flexion pattern of the leg.

Movement

Having used both hands on the foot to obtain stretch and thus initiate the movement, the therapist immediately transfers the hand on the right heel onto the patient's knee giving pressure on the lateral aspect. This encourages both flexion of the knee and abduction of the hip. Care must be taken to keep the knee and foot in line with each other parallel to the resting leg, i.e. the leg is carried across as one piece. If this point is not observed the wrong rotation will occur at the hip. The therapist must ensure that the knee flexion is caused by activity of the hamstrings and not passively by gravity. This is achieved by actively resisting the movement.

The patient moves into medial rotation of the hip, dorsiflexion and eversion of the foot, extension of the toes, knee flexion and flexion and abduction of the hip (Figure 198).

Flexion/abduction/medial rotation with knee extension

Starting position (Figure 199)

PATIENT   To enable the patient to flex the knee of the extended and adducted leg in preparation for knee extension he is moved down the plinth until his knees are level with the foot of the plinth. Both knees can then be flexed. Care must be taken when deciding to use this position as some individuals find that it causes discomfort in the lumbar region even if a pillow is used to support this area. It may be necessary to abandon the normal timing of this pattern and use the Timing for Emphasis technique in the Sitting position.

THERAPIST   *Stance* and *grip* as for the basic pattern. The therapist will need to flex her forward knee more fully to enable her to reach the foot.

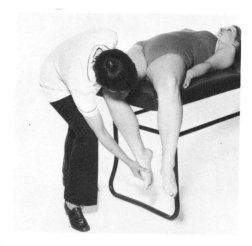

Figure 199   Starting position for the flexion/abduction/medial rotation with knee extension pattern of the leg.

Commands

The basic command is '*now*'—'*pull up and straighten your knee*' although specific instructions, for example '*turn your heel out*', may be necessary.

Movement

Medial rotation of the hip with dorsiflexion and eversion of the foot, extension of the toes, extension of the knee and flexion and abduction of the hip.

Extension/adduction/lateral rotation

Starting position

PATIENT   Flexion/abduction/medial rotation of the hip, dorsiflexion and eversion of the foot and extension of the toes. The resting leg must be abducted to allow the moving leg to come to rest in adduction.

THERAPIST
Stance   The therapist stands in line with the movement diagonal opposite to the patient's hip facing the foot of the plinth with her right foot forwards.
Grip   The therapist places her right hand on the plantar surface of the patient's foot with her thumb under the toes and the heel of her hand giving pressure on the outer border of the foot (Figure 200). Her left hand is placed, approaching from above the leg, on the adductor surface of the thigh with the fingers on the flexor surface of the knee.

Commands

'*Now*'—'*turn your heel in and push your foot down*'. This may be reduced to '*now*'—'*push*'.

Movement

Lateral rotation of the hip, plantarflexion and inversion of the foot, flexion of the toes and extension and adduction of the hip.

In normal timing movement is initiated by the rotary component. Movement then occurs

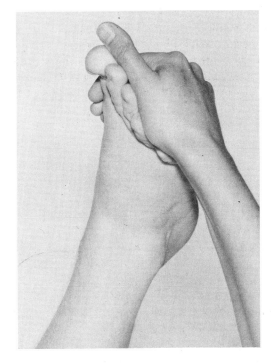

Figure 200   Grip on the foot—starting position for the extension/adduction/lateral rotation pattern of the leg.

at the distal joints to be followed in succession by the more proximal joints. Rotation continues throughout the pattern. The therapist transfers her weight from the rear left foot to the forward right foot and bends the right knee.

Extension/adduction/lateral rotation with knee flexion

Starting position

PATIENT   To accommodate the knee flexion the patient is moved towards the foot end of the plinth until the knees conveniently flex with the patient in Lying. This position, as in the flexion/abduction with the knee extension pattern, may cause discomfort in the lumbar region. In this case it should not be used. The starting position is as for extension/adduction/lateral rotation.

THERAPIST   *Stance* and *grip* as for extension/adduction/lateral rotation except that the left hand is moved proximally away from the knee.

Commands

'*Now*'—'*push*'. Additional commands such as '*bend your knee*' may be used as necessary.

Movement

Lateral rotation of the hip, plantarflexion and inversion of the foot, flexion of the toes, flexion of the knee, extension and adduction of the hip (Figure 201).

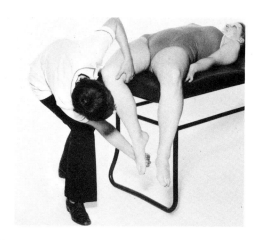

Figure 201   Finishing position for the extension/adduction/lateral rotation with knee flexion pattern of the leg.

Extension/adduction/lateral rotation with knee extension

Starting position

PATIENT   Flexion/abduction/medial rotation of the hip with knee flexion, dorsiflexion and eversion of the foot and extension of the toes.

THERAPIST

Either   *Stance* and *grip* as for extension/adduction/lateral rotation. In this position the therapist is unable to resist a powerful thrust.
Or
Stance   The therapist stands in the Lunge position, right foot forwards, facing the patient on the opposite side of the plinth, i.e. when the patient's right leg is being exercised she stands on the patient's left. In this position she can use her body weight more effectively to give resistance.
Grip   The therapist places her left hand on the plantar surface of the patient's foot so that her fingers are exerting pressure on the patient's toes (Figure 202). The right hand with the thumb abducted is placed on the posterior and

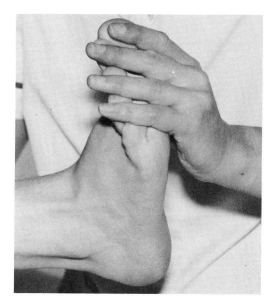

Figure 202   Grip on the foot—alternative starting position for the extension/adduction/lateral rotation with knee extension pattern of the leg.

medial surfaces of the patient's thigh. Initial contact is made with the index finger on the posterior surface and with the thumb on the medial surface. As the movement is executed the thigh 'falls' into the therapist's outstretched hand.

Commands

'*Now*'—'*push*'.

Movement

Lateral rotation of the hip, plantarflexion and inversion of the foot, flexion of the toes, extension of the knee and extension and adduction of the hip. The patient's moving leg crosses the resting leg.

This is the second 'thrust' or 'mass extension' pattern of the lower limb.

CHAPTER 24

P.N.F Head and Neck; Scapular; and Trunk Patterns

P. J. WADDINGTON

HEAD AND NECK PATTERNS

As with the limb patterns, each head and neck pattern has three components resulting in a diagonal movement. These are rotation either to the right or left most of which takes place at the atlanto-axial joint and either flexion or extension at two levels, i.e. at the atlanto-occipital joint only, a nodding movement of the head on the neck, and the second a large movement involving in addition the whole of the cervical vertebrae.

Care must be taken to ensure that rotation occurs throughout the whole movement. If full rotation is allowed to occur too soon ex-

tension and flexion will be limited and the movement will not be in a diagonal direction. This diagonal is in line with the oblique muscles of the trunk. The therapist may ask the patient to look at the hand in the extension/adduction/medial rotation position to give the inner range position of the flexed and rotated head and neck and ask the patient to look at the hand in the flexion/abduction/lateral rotation position to give the inner range position of the extended and rotated head and neck. The chin will be seen to move in a straight line in a diagonal direction.

Extension with rotation to the right

Starting position (Figure 203)

PATIENT Supine with the shoulders level with the end of the plinth. Flexion of the head with rotation to the left.

THERAPIST

Stance The therapist stands at the head end of the plinth in the Lunge position with the right leg forwards.

Grip The therapist places the thumb of her right hand on the lateral surface of the right half of the mandible. The rest of the hand and fingers are kept well away from contact with the patient.

The left hand is placed, thumb abducted

with fingers down, on the occiput. The temptation to put this hand near to the nape of the neck must be resisted as the wrist will be placed in an uncomfortable position when the patient moves into extension.

Commands

'*Now*'—'*push and look to the right*'.

Movement

Extension of the head and neck with rotation to the right (Figure 204).

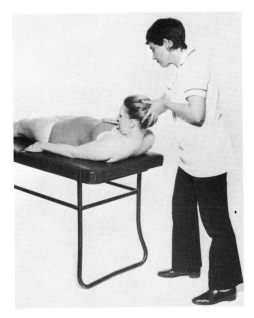

Figure 203 Neck patterns—starting position for extension with rotation to the right.

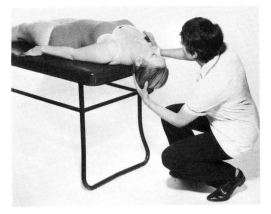

Figure 204 Neck patterns—finishing position for extension with rotation to the right.

Flexion with rotation to the right

Starting position (Figure 205)

PATIENT   Lying with the shoulders level with the edge of the plinth. Extension of the head and neck with rotation to the left.

THERAPIST

Stance   As for extension with rotation to the right, but with the left foot forward.

Grip   The therapist may choose to use either hand on the chin and vice versa on the occiput but it is convenient to use the left hand on the mandible so that the slow reversal technique (Chapter 25) may be used.

The little and ring fingers of the left hand are placed on the inferior border of the right half of the mandible. If more fingers are used there is a tendency to press on the patient's larynx and cause discomfort.

The right hand is on the occiput as for extension with rotation to the left.

Commands

'*Now*'—'*pull your chin up towards your breast pocket*'.

Movement

Flexion of the head and neck with rotation to the right (Figure 206).

Head and neck patterns can usefully be done with the patient in Forearm Support Prone Lying either on the plinth or on the mat. It may also be found to be of value to use the extensor patterns with the patient in the

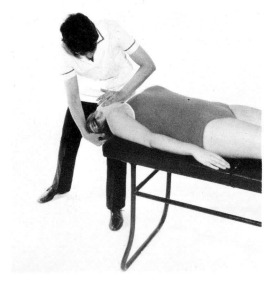

Figure 205 Neck patterns—starting position for flexion with rotation to the right.

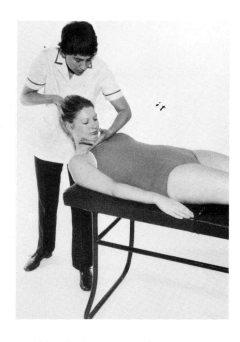

Figure 206 Neck patterns—finishing position for flexion with rotation to the right.

Sitting position. This will assist the patient to gain a good position of the head and thus favourably affect posture in general.

Using the Timing for Emphasis technique (Chapter 25) and the head and neck as the 'handle', the strong neck muscles can be used to obtain a contraction of the abdominal muscles (flexion with rotation) and the erector spinae (extension with rotation).

SHOULDER GIRDLE OR SCAPULAR PATTERNS

Each scapular pattern has three components: either elevation or depression, either abduction (protraction) or adduction (retraction) and rotation round the chest wall (Figure 207).

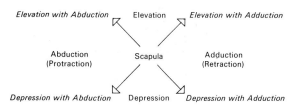

Figure 207 Diagram showing the diagonal movements of the scapula.

It will be noted that the terms abduction and adduction are used instead of the more usual protraction and retraction. This is quite logical as the protracted scapula has been moved away from the central axis of the body, i.e. into abduction; and the retracted scapula has been moved towards the central axis, i.e. into adduction.

Elevation with abduction

Starting position

PATIENT The patient is placed either on the plinth or on the mat in Side Lying with hips and knees flexed sufficiently to give stability. Care must be taken not to allow the patient to assume a semi-prone position.

THERAPIST

Stance The therapist Stands or Kneels behind the patient in line with the movement diagonal, i.e. near to the patient's hips.

Grip The therapist places her left hand on the point of the patient's shoulder and exerts stretch by pulling the shoulder into depression and adduction, i.e. towards the left hip. She may use her right hand to support her left hand or to control the patient's arm.

Commands

'*Now*'—'*pull up towards your nose*'.

Movement

Elevation and abduction of the scapula with rotation round the chest wall. This movement is associated with the flexion/adduction/lateral rotation pattern of the arm.

Depression with abduction

Starting position

PATIENT As for elevation with abduction.

THERAPIST

Stance The therapist Stands or Kneels behind the patient in line with the movement diagonal, i.e. near to the patient's head.

Grip As for elevation with abduction except that the pressure is such that it stimulates the movement required. The therapist exerts stretch by pulling the shoulder into elevation and adduction, i.e. towards the nape of the patient's neck.

Commands

'*Now*'—'*pull down towards your left hip*'.

Movement

Depression and abduction of the scapula with rotation round the chest wall. This movement is associated with the extension/adduction/medial rotation pattern of the arm.

Note for both abduction patterns of the scapula the therapist positions herself behind the patient.

Elevation with adduction

Starting position

PATIENT As for elevation with abduction.

THERAPIST

Stance The therapist Stands or Kneels in front of the patient in line with the movement diagonal, i.e. near to the patient's hip.

Grip The therapist places both hands usually left on top of right on the scapula with her fingers round the medial border. She exerts stretch by pulling the shoulder into depression and abduction, i.e. towards the patient's left hip.

Commands

'*Now*'—'*pull up towards the back of your neck*'.

Movement

Elevation and adduction of the scapula with rotation round the chest wall. This movement is associated with the flexion/abduction/lateral rotation pattern of the arm.

Depression with adduction

Starting position

PATIENT   As for elevation with abduction.

THERAPIST

Stance The therapist Stands or Kneels in front of the patient in line with the movement diagonal, i.e. near to the patient's head.

Grip As for elevation with adduction except that the pressure is such that it stimulates the movement required. The therapist exerts stretch by pulling the shoulder into elevation and abduction, i.e. towards the patient's nose.

Commands

'*Now*'—'*pull down towards your left hip*'.

Movement

Depression and adduction of the scapula with rotation round the chest wall. This movement is associated with the extension/abduction/medial rotation pattern of the arm.

Scapular patterns are important in two specific areas of rehabilitation.

1   Correct movement of the scapula is vital for normal functioning of the upper limb.

2   Strong movements of the scapula working in pattern may be used to facilitate rolling activities on mats.

PELVIC GIRDLE PATTERNS

There are four movements of the pelvis in line with and exercising the oblique abdominal muscles.

Pelvic girdle patterns are usually done in Side Lying on the mat where the patient feels more secure and where they can be used as a means of teaching rolling.

The therapist Kneels at one end of the diagonal line of movement behind the patient. She grasps the iliac crest using this as a 'handle' to obtain stretch and give resistance to the forward movements of the pelvis. For the backwards movements of the pelvis the therapist presses with the heel of one hand supported by the other hand on the ischial tuberosity.

TRUNK PATTERNS
Using the head and neck and arms
Flexion with rotation (chopping)

Starting position for rotation to the right

PATIENT   The patient is in Lying. His right arm is placed in the position of flexion/adduction/lateral rotation. He grasps his right wrist with his left hand. His forearm is supinated.

The patient is instructed to look at his right

hand thus assuming the head and neck position of extension with rotation to the left.

THERAPIST

Stance The therapist is on the patient's right at the side of the plinth in the Lunge position with her left foot forwards facing the patient's head, as for the extension/abduction/medial rotation pattern of the arm.

Grip The therapist uses her right hand to grasp the patient's right hand as for the extension/abduction/medial rotation pattern of the arm. She places her left hand, as if she were pushing, over the near part of the patient's forehead.

Commands

'Now'—'push'.

Movement

The head and neck move into flexion with rotation to the right. The right arm moves into extension/abduction/medial rotation of the shoulder, pronation of the forearm, extension of the wrist and fingers with abduction of the thumb and the left arm moves in a supporting role. The trunk is flexed and rotated to the right (Figure 208).

The Timing for Emphasis technique (Chapter 25) may be used here to strengthen

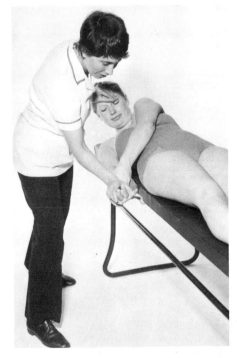

Figure 208 Finishing position for 'Chopping' to the right.

the abdominal muscles with the head and neck and the arms used as the 'handle' held in inner range and using the lumbar spine as the 'pivot'. For the average individual very little resistance will prove to be maximal.

Extension with rotation (lifting)

Starting position as for rotation to the right

PATIENT The patient is Supine with his shoulders level with the top of the plinth. His right arm is placed in the position of extension/adduction/medial rotation. He grasps his right wrist with his left hand, with supinated forearm. The patient is instructed to look at his right

hand thus assuming the head and neck position of flexion with rotation to the left.

THERAPIST

Stance The therapist is on the patient's right at the side of the plinth in the Lunge position with her right foot forwards facing the patient's feet. She should be as near to the patient's head as possible while still able to reach his right hand with her right hand. Her reach will be increased by flexing her right knee.

Grip   The therapist grasps the patient's right hand with her right hand. On this occasion the thumb and not the fingers will be in a position to resist the rotation of the upper limb. She places her left hand on the crown of the patient's head, fingers towards the nape of his neck.

Commands

'*Keep looking at your hand*', '*now*'—'*push*'.

Movement

The head and neck move into extension with rotation to the right. The right arm moves into flexion/abduction/lateral rotation of the shoulder, supination of the forearm, extension of the wrist, fingers and thumb. The left arm

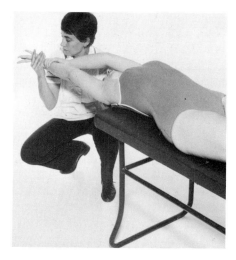

Figure 209   Finishing position for 'Lifting' to the right.

moves in a supporting role. The trunk is extended and rotated to the right (Figure 209).

Using the legs

The basic patterns of the legs are used as a means of obtaining trunk movement. In these patterns both legs move simultaneously keeping together throughout the movement. Thus they move in asymmetrical patterns; for example, for the left leg to remain with the right leg throughout the flexion/adduction/lateral rotation pattern, it will have to move into flexion/abduction/medial rotation.

Flexion with rotation (straight knees)

Starting position as for rotation to the left

PATIENT   The patient is in Supine close to his right-hand side of the plinth.

The right leg is in extension, abduction, medial rotation of the hip, plantarflexion and eversion of the foot and flexion of the toes. The left leg is in extension, adduction, lateral rotation of the hip, plantarflexion and inversion of the foot and flexion of the toes.

THERAPIST
Stance   The therapist stands facing the patient on his right side in the Lunge position in a diagonal direction with her left foot forwards and slightly proximal to the level of the patient's feet.
Grip   The therapist places her right hand on the dorsum of both of the patient's feet and her left hand and forearm are placed on the anterior aspect of the patient's thigh near to

the knees. If the patient has difficulty in lifting his legs the therapist may place her left fore-arm underneath the patient's knees supporting his legs while the hand is in contact with the lateral surface of the patient's left thigh.

Commands

'*Now*'—'*turn your heels away from me—pull up*'. The patient may need to be reminded to dorsiflex the feet.

Movement

The legs move as one. The right leg into flexion/adduction/lateral rotation of the hip, dorsiflexion and inversion of the foot with extension of the toes. The left leg moves into flexion/abduction/medial rotation of the hip, dorsiflexion and inversion of the foot with extension of the toes. This is followed by flexion of the trunk with rotation to the left.

This is a very difficult exercise and with the average patient it will be noted that the pull of psoas major and iliacus will have an adverse effect on the lumbar spine and pelvic tilt, causing extension of the lumbar spine to occur.

The same pattern but with knee flexion will be found to be strong enough for the vast majority of patients (Figure 210). The Timing for Emphasis technique (Chapter 25) is of value here. The legs, with flexed knees, form the 'handle' and the lumbar spine is the 'pivot'. A series of Repeated Contractions done

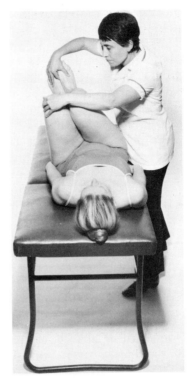

Figure 210   Finishing position for the double leg, hip and knee flexion pattern.

in this way is valuable for strengthening the abdominal muscles.

The pattern starting with the knees flexed and finishing with the knees in extension may also be used but again the therapist and patient may experience the same problems with the lumbar spine and pelvic tilt as in the straight leg pattern.

Extension with rotation (straight knees)

This is a valuable pattern for facilitating back extension.

Starting position for rotation to the right

PATIENT   The patient is in Supine close to his right-hand side of the plinth. The right leg is in flexion/adduction/lateral rotation of the hip, dorsiflexion and inversion of the foot and extension of the toes. The left leg is in flexion/abduction/medial rotation of the hip, dorsiflexion and eversion of the foot and extension of the toes.

The therapist may have to assist the patient into the starting position.

THERAPIST

Stance   The therapist stands on the patient's right at the side of the plinth, in the Lunge position with her left foot forward facing the patient's head. The therapist must stand close to the patient with her elbows tucked into her body so that the force of the patient's effort is transmitted as directly as possible, through her straight back, to the floor.

Grip   The therapist places her right hand on the plantar surface of the patient's feet with her thumb as far as possible under his toes in a position to resist flexion. The therapist places the left forearm under the patient's legs at above the level of his knees.

Commands

'*Now*'—'*turn your heels towards me and push down*'.

Movement

The legs move as one, the right leg into extension, abduction, medial rotation of the hip with plantarflexion and eversion of the foot and flexion of the toes and the left leg into extension, adduction and lateral rotation of the hip with plantarflexion and inversion of the foot and flexion of the toes.

Knee extension

This is probably the strongest movement available to an individual, i.e. thrusting with both legs. The therapist must be able to control the patient and care must be exercised in selecting suitable patients. It may be used when one leg is reasonably strong and the other weak. The therapist uses 'overflow' from the stronger leg to facilitate activity in the weaker. It may also be used to gain general extension in the very weak patient.

The pattern and positioning are the same as for the straight knee pattern except that the patient starts with his knees flexed.

Knee flexion

This pattern may be used to facilitate back extension. The pattern and positioning are the same as for the straight knee pattern except that the patient finishes the movement with flexed knees.

Side flexion (quadratus lumborum pattern using the legs)

Side flexion of the trunk to produce a 'hip hitching' movement is valuable but sometimes difficult to teach a patient. It can be achieved easily by applying P.N.F. principles.

Starting position for left side flexion (Figure 211)

PATIENT   The patient is placed in Lying on a plinth with his heels minimally over the end of the plinth.

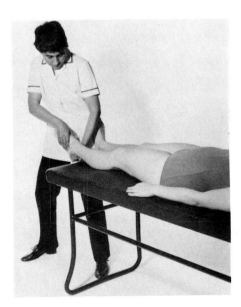

Figure 211 Starting position for trunk side flexion to the left.

onto her left hip giving enough pressure to keep his leg straight in that position.

Grip The therapist places her left hand under the patient's left heel and her right hand on the dorsum of his foot near to the ankle. She then pulls down with both hands in the direction of the long axis of the leg. Care must be taken to pull equally with both hands. Too much pressure with the right hand will force the foot into plantarflexion. This should be avoided.

Commands

'*Now*'—'*pull up*'.

Movement

The patient side flexes by hitching his hip and in effect 'shortening' his left leg.

A quick gentle stretch will initiate the stretch reflex and result in contraction and movement. The therapist must be careful to allow the movement to take place as such a contraction is weak. The maximal resistance principle together with Repeated Contractions (Chapter 25) may be used as a strengthening technique.

THERAPIST

Stance The therapist stands at the foot of the plinth in the Lunge position with her left foot forwards. She places the patient's right foot

OTHER CONSIDERATIONS

P.N.F. principles can be applied to exercises for the respiratory muscles, the muscles of the face and jaw, and, by using a wooden tongue depressor, exercises can be given to the tongue and the buccinator muscles.

Stimulation round the face and mouth can be very valuable as these areas are well supplied with sensory receptors.

MECHANICAL LOADING

Progressive resistance exercises using pulley and weight circuits form a part of many treatment programmes. When viewed from the neurophysiological standpoint exercises done against mechanical resistance cannot be considered to be as effective as those done against manual resistance. The features associated with the expert grip of the therapist are absent.

1 Precise exteroceptive stimulation.
2 Stretch stimulus.

3 Graduated resistance ensuring the patient's maximum effort through full range.

However, a pulley and weight circuit may form a useful part of an intensive treatment programme. It is valuable in increasing the patient's exercise tolerance and the therapist can supervise a small group of patients. This may have the beneficial effect of reducing the patient's dependence upon the therapist which can develop in a one-to-one situation.

It is possible to arrange such circuits so that the patient is working in pattern by positioning him so that the rope is in the line of the diagonal on completion of the movement. All patterns may be done in this way (Figure 212).

The main aim of a mechanically resisted programme when used in conjunction with manually resisted exercises is to improve the patient's endurance. It is therefore advisable to give low resistance so that a high number of repetitions is necessary for maximum effort.

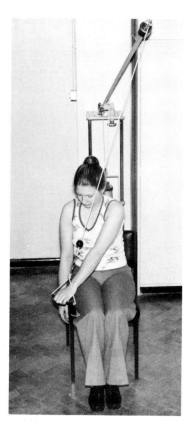

Figure 212 Using a weight and pulley circuit to resist the extension/adduction/medial rotation pattern of the arm.

CHAPTER 25

P.N.F. Techniques

P. J. WADDINGTON

In therapeutic exercise coordinated patterns of movement facilitated by the correct sensory input must be augmented by specific techniques of emphasis.

Basically these fall into the two fundamental categories, muscle strengthening and joint mobilizing techniques. Although it is theoretically and practically convenient to conceive the problems presented by patients in this way, therapists are well aware that the two are indivisible although certain techniques are much more effective in strengthening muscles and others in increasing the range of movement.

STRENGTHENING TECHNIQUES

There are two main techniques which may be used for strengthening: *Repeated Contractions*; and *Slow Reversals*.

Repeated contractions

There are three variations of this technique.

Normal timing

This is probably the simplest of all the techniques once the patterns have been learned.

It consists of repeating any chosen pattern several times through full range against maximum resistance ensuring smooth movement at all times. As with other methods of applying progressive resistance exercises the therapist may determine the relationship between the amount of resistance and the number of repetitions.

The therapist selects the pattern or patterns in which the muscle to be strengthened works to advantage and the patient moves through full range. Once the pattern has been completed, i.e. the muscles are in their shortened range, the therapist passively returns the limb to the lengthened position ready for the next repetition.

The firing of motor units is prolonged due to bombardment of the motor neurons by many impulses (summation). This prolongation of the response is called 'after discharge'.

Timing for Emphasis

This is a technique in which the Irradiation/Overflow principle is used to facilitate the contraction of a weak group of muscles.

The patient's strong muscles maximally contracting facilitate the contraction of a weaker group through recruitment. This 'overflow' principle can be used from one limb to another or from the head or limbs to the trunk or vice versa. The therapist must analyse the patient's strengths and weaknesses as overflow is only effective from strong to weak muscles. 'Timing for Emphasis' is the method by which this overflow principle is applied to the muscles within a single pattern. For example, a weak deltoid muscle may be strengthened by exercising it in two patterns, i.e. flexion/abduction with lateral rotation and extension/abduction with medial rotation. The fundamental feature of Timing for Emphasis is that the other muscles in the pattern are made to contract maximally to facilitate the contraction of the weak muscle while movement is allowed only in one joint or in the case of the elbow, movement is also allowed in the radioulnar joints.

It is natural for an individual to make every effort to complete a movement.

A pattern used in this manner is described as having three parts: 1, *pivot*; 2, *handle*; 3, *stabilizing part*.

Pivot   The pivot is the joint in which movement is taking place. This movement is brought about by the weak muscles.

Handle   The handle is the part the therapist is holding, distal to the pivot. The strong muscles in this part of the pattern are contracting in inner range.

Stabilizing part   This is the part of the pattern proximal to the pivot controlled by strong muscles. The muscles here are usually contracting in middle range.

There are two methods by which this can be achieved.

a   The therapist may prevent the patient from moving in any part of the pattern except over the pivot, i.e. the patient is prevented from further contracting isotonically by the resistance applied by the therapist.
b   The therapist takes the part passively to the strongest point in the range. The patient is then encouraged to 'hold' at that point, i.e. to

perform an isometric contraction and then movement is allowed at the pivot.

The wrist flexors may be used as another example. Flexion of the wrist towards the radial side takes place in the flexion/adduction/lateral rotation pattern with elbow flexion and supination. The pattern is allowed to proceed or the limb is taken to a point in the range where the proximal components are in middle range and the distal components, the flexors of the fingers, are contracting in inner range. Further movement ceases except in the wrist joint where movement is allowed and the range completed. The therapist, while maintaining the position of the rest of the pattern, returns the wrist to the extended position and the patient is encouraged to repeat the movement. Thus the normal timing sequence has been changed to emphasize the contraction of the weak component, i.e. the wrist flexors—especially flexor carpi radialis. This group is then subjected to a form of 'Repeated Contractions' facilitated by the other strong muscles in the pattern working maximally.

In this example the flexors, adductors and lateral rotators of the glenohumeral joint, the flexors of the elbow and supinators form the *stabilizing part*, the wrist joint is the *pivot* and the flexors of the fingers and adductor of the thumb constitute the *handle*. The therapist's grip is that used in the basic pattern.

When learning and exploring the possibilities of this technique the therapist may choose to analyse the movements and muscles involved in two ways.

1   By taking each pattern the therapist may allow movement to occur in successive pivots, i.e. glenohumeral, elbow, wrist, etc., or hip, knee, ankle, etc. For example: flexion/adduction/lateral rotation with knee extension; grip as for basic pattern (Table 1).

Table 1

Pivot	Starting position	Movement	Muscles subjected to repeated contraction
Hip	Supine Lying, *Hip* flexed and adducted in the part of the range selected for strengthening—this is frequently middle or inner range. *Knee* flexed in middle range (care must be taken to ensure that the patient is actively contracting his hamstring muscles). *Ankle and foot* dorsiflexed, inverted, toes extended in inner range	Flexion, adduction, lateral rotation	Hip flexors—psoas major, iliacus, rectus femoris (acting over the hip), Hip adductors and lateral rotators—adductor brevis, adductor longus, gracilis, pectineus and the small lateral rotator muscles
Knee	Either Supine Lying or Sitting over the side of the plinth. *Hip* flexed and adducted in middle range. *Knee* flexed in preparation for extension in the part of the range selected for strengthening. *Ankle and foot* dorsiflexed, inverted, toes extended in inner range	Extension of the knee	Vastus medialis and rectus femoris (medial component)
Ankle and talocalcaneonavicular joint	Any starting position although Supine Lying is frequently convenient. *Hip* flexed and adducted in middle range. *Knee*, the therapist has to decide whether she requires flexion or extension—she must consider two major factors: the length of and/or tone of gastrocnemius and, that the functional combination of movements in walking is dorsiflexion with knee extension. *Ankle and foot* plantarflexed and everted in preparation for movement, toes extended	Dorsiflexion and inversion	Tibilais anterior

2 The therapist may prefer to analyse the movement and muscle work occurring at each joint in all four patterns before moving on to the next joint. For example: A, the wrist (**Figure 213**); B, the thumb (**Figure 214**).

Combining isotonic and isometric muscle work (Figure 215)

This method is designed to strengthen a muscle in a specific part of the range and is of particular value in strengthening a muscle following

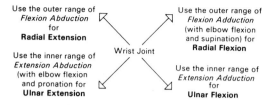

Figure 213 Diagrammatic representation of the movements occurring at the wrist in the four basic arm patterns; giving the range in which the best results may be obtained when using the Timing for Emphasis technique.

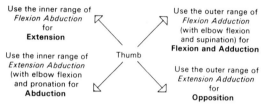

Figure 214 Diagrammatic representation of the movements occurring at the thumb in the four basic arm patterns; giving the range in which the best results may be obtained when using the Timing for Emphasis technique.

an increase in the range of movement, e.g. when treating a frozen shoulder.

The therapist's aim is to facilitate the isotonic contraction of muscles which have not been active for some time in this shortened range.

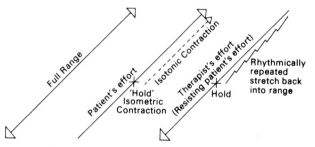

Figure 215 Diagrammatic representation of the strengthening technique combining isotonic and isometric muscle work.

Take the limb either passively or actively to a strong part of the range adjacent to the range selected for strengthening. The patient is then instructed to '*hold*' and a maximal isometric contraction of the agonists is developed at this point where the muscles are strong. The patient is then instructed to '*push*' or '*pull*', i.e. to endeavour to complete full range—the muscles working isotonically.

The therapist then rhythmically and repeatedly rotates the limb a short distance into the antagonist pattern; each time giving the contracting muscle a gentle stretch to stimulate further muscle contraction.

This method also aids the relaxation or lengthening reaction of the antagonist group (reciprocal innervation) by facilitation of the contraction of the agonists, thus assisting in maintaining the increased range previously gained.

Slow Reversal

In this technique the contraction of the strong muscles in the antagonist pattern is used to facilitate the contraction of the weaker muscles of the agonist group. The basis for the slow reversal technique is Sherrington's Principle of Successive Induction. Sherrington noted that immediately the flexor reflex had been elicited the excitability of the extensor reflex was increased.

When the therapist is applying the 'Slow Reversal' technique she uses the maximal contraction of the stronger antagonist group to facilitate the contraction of the weaker agonist group.

For example, to strengthen deltoid in the flexion/abduction/lateral rotation pattern the patient is instructed to complete the extension/adduction/medial rotation pattern. The therapist ensures that the patient is working maximally. On completion of the movement the therapist, smoothly and without pause, changes her grip and the patient moves into the flexion/abduction/lateral rotation pattern. The sequence is then repeated several times.

RELAXATION/LENGTHENING TECHNIQUES

There are two methods by which the therapist may endeavour to obtain a lengthening re-action of the antagonist group, hypertonus of which is preventing the patient from moving further into the agonist pattern.

1 Working the hypertonic group

The therapist elicits a maximal contraction of the antagonist group ensuring that the maximum number of motor units is contracting simultaneously. Following the contraction the muscle will relax and the therapist takes advantage of the relaxation to move the part further into the agonist range. The more motor units the therapist can facilitate to contract together the better the result, as all these motor units will also relax simultaneously.

There are two techniques which take advantage of this physiological fact: *Contract Relax*; and *Hold Relax*.

The fundamental difference between these techniques is the type of muscle contraction. Contract Relax uses an isotonic contraction of the antagonists and Hold Relax, as the name implies, uses an isometric contraction.

Contract Relax

The therapist takes the part passively or resists the active movement of the part to the point where further movement into the agonist pattern is limited by tension in the antagonist group. She then changes her grip to that used for the antagonist pattern and instructs the patient to '*pull*' or '*push*'. By her resistance the therapist only allows the patient to move a short way into rotation, preventing movement from occurring in the other components of the pattern. When the therapist is sure that the patient is working maximally she instructs him to '*relax*' and then she gradually relaxes her resistance while maintaining her grip. Time is then allowed for relaxation to occur. The therapist then changes her grip carefully and moves the part gently further into the agonist pattern. The process can be repeated at the point where resistance to further movement is experienced.

Hold Relax

As for Contract Relax the therapist takes the limb to the point where further movement into the agonist pattern is prevented by tension in the antagonists. This movement may be passive or active. The therapist smoothly changes to the grip for the antagonist pattern and instructs the patient to '*hold*' slowly, by concentrating on the rotary component, the therapist builds up the resistance until the patient is contracting his muscles maximally. The therapist must never break or overcome the patient's maximal isometric contraction. The patient is instructed to '*relax*' and the sequence completed as for the Contract Relax technique.

Advantages and disadvantages Hold Relax is frequently the technique of choice. The slow build up and isometric contraction ensures that there is no joint movement and when the problem is one of pain the lack of movement will ensure that the patient is relatively pain-free. Pain is counter productive as it will increase the unwanted hypertonus.

The other advantage of Hold Relax is that when treating a particularly strong patient the therapist maintains control of the situation. If she were to allow movement the patient might be able to overcome her resistance.

The advantage of Contract Relax is that in some situations the patient may find it is difficult to perform an isometric contraction.

2 Working the reciprocal group (to the hypertonic group)

Contraction of a muscle is accompanied by relaxation of the antagonist group.

Slow Reversal—Hold Relax

The method for the Hold Relax technique is used until the point when the patient is told to relax, i.e. the patient is taken actively or passively to the point where limitation occurs, he is then instructed to contract in the direction of tightness, this is followed by relaxation. The therapist then changes her grip to the reverse pattern. The patient moves further into the previously restricted range (isotonic contraction) against maximal resistance. This technique thus uses both approaches to obtaining the lengthening reaction. This method is particularly valuable when the agonist group of muscles is strong.

Reciprocal lengthening reaction

Although it is not included as a P.N.F. technique the therapist can obtain a reciprocal lengthening reaction of a group of muscles in spasm (the antagonists) by causing the agonist group to contract isometrically against maximal resistance at the point of limitation.

This method is particularly successful when trying to increase the range of movement at the knee joint, when further flexion is prevented by the failure of the quadriceps to lengthen due to spasm. The therapist gains relaxation by causing the hamstrings to contract maximally. Overflow may be used by maximally resisting the contraction of the hamstring group of the uninjured leg. The patient is positioned in Sitting over the side of the plinth and the therapist sits on the floor. The therapist gives resistance to the hamstrings by grasping the plantar surfaces of the patient's feet; thus activating the gastrocnemius (a knee flexor) and the other plantarflexors as well.

Additional techniques

Rhythmic stabilization

This technique is based on isometric muscle work where there is a simultaneous isometric contraction of all muscles controlling the joint. The result is called co-contraction.

'Rhythmic Stabilization' can be used either to gain relaxation or increase strength.

Relaxation The part is taken to the point where limitation occurs. The therapist gives the command '*hold*'. Emphasizing the rotary component of the pattern the therapist alternates her pressure and thus alternates the resistance between the agonist and antagonist patterns. Gradually the resistance is increased until the patient is working maximally. The therapist must not break the hold. The final '*hold*' is in the pattern antagonistic to the tightness. The patient is then asked to contract isotonically by moving through as much range as possible.

Strength The muscle to be strengthened is

facilitated to contract maximally in the strongest part of the range. At that point the resistance is alternated building up a maximal co-contraction. The final hold is on the side of the muscle to be strengthened and then the patient is instructed to move further into the desired range.

It may take up to 15 minutes after the treatment for the strengthening technique to exhibit its maximum effect.

An additional effect of Rhythmic Stabilization will be to increase the circulation.

Rhythm technique

This technique is applied to the limbs when the patient has difficulty in initiating movement, particularly for patients with Parkinsonism. It is very beneficial when used in conjunction with trunk rotation (as advocated by Mrs Bobath), as relaxation gained centrally affects the peripheral muscles.

The therapist applies the technique to each limb and each pattern in turn.

The therapist takes hold of the patient with a usual grip for the selected pattern. When using this technique with the upper limbs the therapist may find it an advantage to grasp the patient with only the hand which holds the patient's hand, as the two-handed grip tends to impede the rhythmic movement. She begins by passively taking the limb through full range. This is repeated several times until a good rhythm of moderate speed is established. The patient is then instructed to join in gently and assist the movement. Gradually the patient is encouraged to increase his effort ensuring that the tone is not increased. The therapist then repeats the method in the antagonist pattern.

Stretch reflex

The stretch reflex may be used in several ways.

1 The stretch reflex can be used with the 'Repeated Contraction' technique when the extra stretch gives added rhythm to the movement.

2 When the patient cannot move voluntarily a series of stretch reflexes, each followed by the responsive muscle contraction and movement, may be used resulting in a series of repeated contractions. This has value as the patient gets the feeling of movement. He can then try to 'join in'.

3 The stretch reflex can be used to obtain a lengthening reaction

> **a** By obtaining a contraction of the agonist group the antagonist group will reciprocally relax.
>
> **b** A series of contractions of the antagonist (tight) group caused by the therapist applying quick and controlled stretch will result in relaxation or lengthening of the muscle. The therapist gradually takes the limb further into the desired range.

When using stretch reflex the therapist must be sensitive to the resultant movement which is brought about by a relatively weak contraction and allow it to occur. Any appreciable resistance will prevent movement.

CHAPTER 26
Functional Activities on Mats

P. J. WADDINGTON

Functional activities on mats are designed to improve progressively the patient's independence. It is as important to teach the helpless patient to turn in bed as it is to teach re-education of walking to another. The progression of mat activities is based upon the main theme of the normal development sequence, i.e. rolling from Supine to Prone and from Prone to Supine, getting to Prone Kneeling, then to Standing and eventually to gait training. Such activities as teaching the patient to get up from the floor into the Sitting position are also included. These activities are based on the normal patterns of movement but each activity will include more than one pattern. The basic techniques of P.N.F. are applicable to this work. In the actual treatment of a patient, balance activities (Chapter 27) also done for the most part on mats, cannot be divorced from functional activities on mats. As a general rule it is advisable to:

1 *Help* the patient *to take up* a position, e.g. Prone Kneeling, and *teach* him *to retain* that position (power and balance). A patient cannot be expected to attempt with confidence to achieve a position if he believes that he will fall down again once he has gained it.
2 *Teach* the patient *to take up* the position.
3 *Teach* the patient *to move* in the position, e.g. crawl.

Ideally there should be a mat area in the department, the size of which will depend upon the number of patients treated at any one time. Each patient will require a mat at least 1800 × 1740 cm (Low Mat). Mats raised from the floor on a platform 46 cm high (High Mat), i.e. the height of the seat of the average wheelchair, have many advantages particularly when getting a patient onto and off the mat. Patients can also easily be progressed from mat activities to sitting balance on the side of the mat. Ideally a department should have both high and low mats side by side.

The therapist should ensure that people using mats remove their shoes to keep the mats clean.

The basic principles of maximum resistance and the selection of strong patterns to overflow to weaker muscles and movements are the basis of teaching the patient to achieve a specific function. However, it is implicit in these principles that the patient must be allowed to move smoothly through the available range. Therefore, where spasticity is a factor in preventing normal movement inhibition should always precede and accompany movement, which must be at a less voluntary level as voluntary effort will have the effect of potentially increasing tone.

The descriptions and illustrations in this section give the main movements and resistance points which may be used by the therapist. It must be remembered that many more combinations of patterns and techniques, for example Repeated Contractions, may be used by the therapist based on her assessment of each patient's specific needs.

As with balance, it is important for the therapist to observe normal functional movement in others as most of these activities take place at a subconscious level. The individual knows that he has rolled over, that he has got from Lying to Prone Kneeling or to Standing but cannot afterwards describe his movements in detail. This, the therapist must know when faced with the problems of rehabilitation. When conscious control is exerted it is unlikely that the normal individual will achieve such a flowing coordinated movement.

In each section below the main patterns of movement involved in the functional activity will be given.

ROLLING

From Side Lying

If the patient is weak, Side Lying is a good starting position, for very little effort by the patient will result in movement as he is assisted by gravity in either direction. The facilitation of trunk rotation is important when re-educating functional activities. The therapist must position herself in the line of movement, i.e. on the diagonal, as it is very easy to get out of pattern, and thus make the patient's task more difficult. To aid accuracy of pattern and to give some stability to Side Lying as a starting position the patient's knees are flexed.

Scapular patterns

Abduction patterns, particularly the depression/abduction pattern, will cause the model to roll forwards towards the Prone position.

Adduction patterns, particularly the elevation/adduction pattern, will cause the model to roll backwards towards the Supine position.

Pelvic patterns

The patterns are based upon the line and contraction of the oblique abdominal muscle. i.e. from the crest of the ilium and inguinal ligament to the lower ribs of the opposite side. Movement occurs in two directions.

1 Flexion of the trunk with rotation—rolling forwards. The therapist grasps the patient's

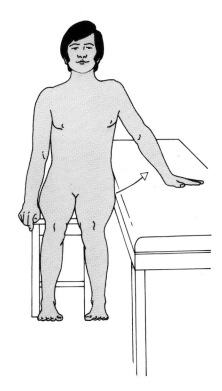

Figure 216 The basic arc of movement used in sideways transfers.

iliac crest near to, and including, the anterior superior iliac spine. Using her body weight by leaning backwards she applies a stretch stimulus. On the command '*now—pull*' the patient moves the pelvis forwards.

2 Extension of the trunk with rotation—rolling backwards. The therapist, using her body weight, gives forward pressure to the patient's pelvis (over gluteus maximus). On the command '*now—push*' the patient moves the pelvis backwards.

This rotation of the pelvis resulting in an arc of movement can be observed in many of the functional activities on mats and in sideways transfer activities, e.g. from chair to bed (Figure 216).

The other basic arc of movement, i.e. in a forwards and backwards or straight movement, can be *observed in* many of the mat and transfer activities, e.g. backwards into a chair drawn up facing the bed (Figure 217).

Scapular and pelvic patterns

A combination of the depression/abduction, scapular pattern and the flexion with rotation, pelvic pattern may be used to teach forward rolling into the Prone position.

A combination of the elevation/adduction scapular pattern and the extension with rotation, pelvic pattern may be used to teach rolling into the Supine position.

As the patient's function improves he can be gradually moved further into either the Supine or the Prone position, thus increasing the range of movement and resistance by gravity. Manual resistance will also be graded to allow for smooth movement throughout the available range.

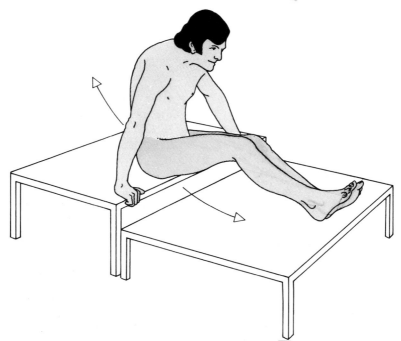

Figure 217 The basic arc of movement used in forwards and backwards transfers.

From Supine to Prone Lying

Most normal individuals when rolling from Supine to Prone use a combination of head and neck, arm and leg patterns. It will be noted that in the majority of instances the head is raised and rotated towards the direction of movement fractionally before the arm and/or leg is moved. Occasionally the normal individual may use mass extension pivoting on the head and heels to initiate a roll. This potentially pathological method should not be encouraged.

The following movements will assist the patient to roll.

Head and neck Flexion with rotation in the direction of movement.

Arm The following methods of using the right arm will cause the patient to roll to the left.

1 Flexion/adduction pattern. The patient

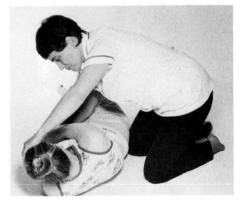

Figure 218 Using the right arm in the extension/adduction position to assist rolling to the left, starting in the Supine position. The therapist may resist the movement using the head and arm.

reaches across his face. He grasps the top edge of the mat or head of the bed and pulls.
2 Extension/adduction pattern. The patient reaches across his body. He grasps the side edge of the mat or bed and pulls (Figure 218).
3 Extension/abduction/elbow extension pattern. The patient places his hand on the mat at waist level and pushes.

The following methods of using the right arm will cause the patient to roll to the right.

1 Flexion/abduction pattern. The patient reaches for the top edge of the mat or bed. He grasps and pulls.
2 Extension/abduction pattern. The patient reaches for the side edge of the mat or bed. He grasps and pulls.

Leg The following methods of using the right leg will assist the patient to roll to the left.

1 The flexion/adduction knee flexion pattern.
2 The extension/abduction/with knee extension pattern. The patient flexes his hip and knee and places his foot on the mat lateral to the mid-line. He thrusts, extending both the hip and the knee.

The following methods of using the right leg will assist the patient to roll to the right.

1 Flexion/abduction pattern either with a straight leg or a flexed knee. The patient should create enough momentum to help his trunk to rotate.
2 Extension/adduction pattern with either a straight leg or extending knee. The patient flexes at the hip and knee (when used) and places the limb in an adducted position. He then pushes with his leg or thrusts his foot into the mat or bed and rolls over.

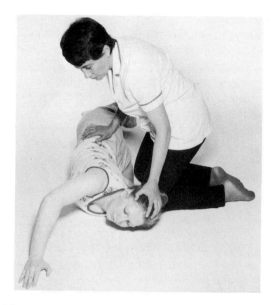

Figure 219   Using the right arm in the flexion/adduction position to assist in rolling to the right starting in the Prone position. The therapist may resist the movement using the head and pelvis.

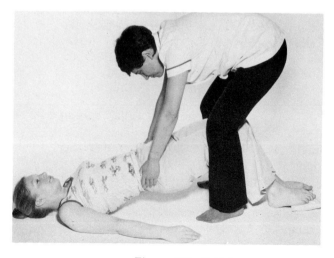

Figure 220   Bridging.

From Prone Lying to Supine

Head   By extending the head and turning it to the right the patient is assisted in rolling to the left.

Arm   By placing the right arm in the following positions with the hand flat on the mat or bed and thrusting, the patient will be assisted in rolling to the left.

1   Flexion/abduction with the elbow flexed sufficiently to allow the palm to be placed on the mat or bed.
2   Extension/abduction with sufficient elbow flexion to allow the palm to be placed on the mat or bed.

By placing the right arm in the position of flexion/adduction with sufficient elbow flexion to allow the palm of the hand to be placed on the mat or bed and thrusting, the patient will be assisted in rolling to the right (Figure 219).

Leg   By raising the right leg backwards, i.e. into the inner range of the extension/adduction pattern, the patient will be assisted in rolling to the left.

BRIDGING

This term denotes pelvic raising from the Crook Lying position. This activity is useful as a preparation for transfers and also for the patient who has to pull clothing over the hips when in Lying. Some patients may find Crook Lying to be a good position from which to initiate rolling.

Before attempting to bridge, the patient must be assisted to maintain the starting position by 'Rhythmic Stabilization' or 'Tapping'.

The therapist positions herself in Standing, facing the patient, with her feet astride his raised knees. She then flexes her hips and knees until she can control the patient's knees with her own knees. It is difficult, in this position, to block the patient's feet as well. If this is necessary a sandbag may be used. The therapist must take care not to strain her back when assisting a patient to bridge.

The therapist places her thumbs inside the waist band of the patient's trousers at the level of the seam. This position enables her, either to resist the patient's bridging activities by pressing on the anterior superior iliac spine or to assist him to lift his hips by taking a firm grip of the trousers and through them to control the pelvis. As the aim is to achieve movement assistance may be necessary initially but the patient should be encouraged to work maximally (Figure 220).

Bridging may be done either sideways with rotation or straight by simply lifting the buttocks straight off the mat. When asking the patient to do the former, the therapist exerts pressure on one anterior superior iliac spine and instructs the patient to raise that hip. He may then return to the starting position or, while in the bridging position, raise first one hip and then the other, thus rotating the pelvis. The therapist gives alternating pressure first on one side and then on the other. For the straight raise pressure is exerted on both hips simultaneously.

Crook Lying is a useful position in which to strengthen the trunk rotators and the hip abductors and adductors.

Trunk rotators

1 The therapist, with her hands in position on the patient's knees, opposite to the proposed direction of movement, instructs the patient to roll the knees towards the mat, first in one direction and then in the other.

Resistance is given to the movement, ensuring that the patient is working maximally.
2 With the patient in the bridging position, i.e. pelvis raised, the therapist uses the 'Rhythmic Stabilization' technique working on the rotators. The therapist's hands are placed one over the anterior superior iliac spine and the other on the opposite buttock. The hands are thus in a position to exert pressure in a rotatory direction. They then alternate.

Hip abductors and adductors

The therapist places each of her hands on the lateral aspect of the appropriate knee. She then resists the movement of abduction with lateral rotation. She then places her hands on the medial aspect of the abducted knees and resists adduction with medial rotation (to midline).

CREEPING

This term denotes either forward or backward progression in either Prone Lying or Forearm Support Prone Lying.

The more primitive form of creeping is an ipsilateral (amphibian) movement of the head, trunk, arm and leg. Later this may develop into the more mature contralateral movement.

Starting position

As the individual's mode of progression matures he will gradually raise his head more and assume the Forearm Support Prone Lying position.

In preparation for this activity, the patient may be placed in the Forearm Support Prone Lying position. The patient rolls into Prone Lying and the therapist stands astride his thorax facing towards his head. To raise the patient onto his right elbow the therapist places her left hand under the patient's shoulder girdle (clavicle) and lifts his shoulder off the mat. With her right hand she positions the patient's arm ensuring that his elbow is directly below the point of the shoulder. Any deviation from this exact position will cause instability. To retain the elbow in the correct position, the therapist fixes it with her right foot. The same method is used to position the patient's left elbow.

'Rhythmic Stabilization' using the head and/or shoulder or 'Tapping' on the shoulders may be used to teach the patient to maintain the position.

The patient is then taught to get into this position unaided.

Movement

Creeping forwards   The therapist takes up a position behind the patient, grasps the feet and resists the forward movement of the leg as it flexes and abducts with lateral rotation. The patient is then instructed to move the arm into flexion/abduction and to turn his head towards the moving limbs.

Progress is made by alternate total flexion on one side and then on the other.

Creeping backwards   Reverse movements cause the individual to progress backwards.

Other activities

The Forearm Support position is useful to enable the patient to learn early control of the head. The 'Rhythmic Stabilization' technique may be used. 'Repeated Contraction' and 'Slow Reversal' techniques, working in the neck flexion and extension patterns can be successfully done in this position as a means of strengthening weak muscles.

Where the neck muscles are strong they may be used in accordance with the overflow principle to strengthen weaker back extensor and abdominal muscles.

CRAWLING

It is not necessary, particularly with adult patients, always to progress through creeping to crawling. Crawling can be attempted as the first mode of progression. To achieve crawling the patient is taken through several stages.

Starting position

Forearm Support Prone Lying   See above.

Forearm Support Prone Kneeling   The patient takes up the Forearm Support Prone Lying position. The therapist stands astride him at hip level facing the patient's head. Bending at the hips and knees, she inserts her thumbs into the waist band of the patient's trousers and grasps the pelvis. She then lifts and raises his pelvis well clear of the mat. The patient's knees are either positioned under the raised hips or the hips are taken slightly backwards over the knees. The patient's knees are abducted a little to ensure a stable position. The therapist's knees which are on either side of the pelvis can, if necessary, control the patient's buttocks.

The patient then learns to balance in this position.

Prone Kneeling   From the Forearm Support Prone Kneeling position the patient is raised into Prone Kneeling. The therapist raises the patient's right shoulder by placing her left hand over the clavicle from behind and uses her right hand to support the patient's right elbow as she lowers his weight onto his outstretched hand. If the patient cannot fully extend the wrist and fingers some adjustment can be made, for example, the hand may be placed on a sandbag. This enables the patient to place weight through the upper limb and to establish the *positive support reaction* (protective extension reaction). In some situations the patient may find it helpful to take his weight through his knuckles. This has the effect of elongating the arm, thus causing the elbow to flex and giving a better position for weight bearing and a thrust.

To free her hands to position the patient's left arm the therapist may have to support his right elbow with her knee.

In this description the right arm has been positioned first; in practice if the patient has one arm which functions better than the other, that arm will be positioned first or the therapist may raise both shoulders simultaneously by placing her hands one over each clavicle and lifting.

The patient then learns to balance in the position.

Teaching the patient to achieve the starting position

There are two basic ways for an individual to achieve Prone Kneeling.

Through Side Sitting From Prone Lying the patient raises his head, places one or both hands flat on the floor beneath his shoulder/s and thrusts. Simultaneously he rotates his trunk and pushes himself into Side Sitting. When one hand is used the patient rotates towards and sits to that side.

From the Supine Position the patient raises his head rotating it towards the stronger side. Almost simultaneously he raises the opposite shoulder (depression/abduction), rotates his trunk and raises himself up to rest on his forearm. The knees are flexed and the pelvis rotated in the same direction. The patient then pushes on his forearm and hand until he has achieved Side Sitting supported by the extended upper limb. With one or both hands on the mat he thrusts on his hands and knees and raises his pelvis sideways in an arc of movement.

To train the patient to do this the therapist places the patient in the Prone Kneeling position and kneels at one side of him. If the patient has weakness down one side the therapist will kneel at the stronger side.

The therapist grasps the patient's waist band and pulls his pelvis slightly towards herself. The patient is then instructed to '*pull up*' and applying the maximal resistance principle, the therapist allows him to regain the Prone Kneeling position (Figure 221).

The therapist gradually moves herself into the Kneel Sitting position, so that each time the patient will be pulled further towards the

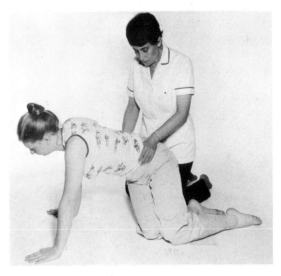

Figure 221 Teaching the patient to achieve Prone Kneeling from Side Sitting.

Side Sitting position and he will have to raise his pelvis through a larger arc of movement to return to Prone Kneeling. Finally, the patient raises his own pelvis from Side Sitting on the mat.

The advantage of the therapist working from the stronger side will now be obvious, i.e. the patient is able to use the stronger (underneath) arm and leg to thrust himself from the floor. The therapist may decide that it is to the patient's advantage to teach him to do the movement from both sides.

Movement backwards from Prone Lying prior to which the patient places his hands under his shoulders. He will either extend his neck in mid-line or extend and rotate the head to one side as he thrusts backwards with his arms and bends his hips and knees.

In practice it will be noted that it is usually the younger people, or those with good power in both arms who use this method.

To emphasize the movement the therapist gives resistance with one hand to the extensors and rotators of the neck by placing one hand on the head opposite to the direction of move-ment and with the other hand placed over the opposite scapula.

In preparation for crawling the patient learns to balance both in the basic Prone Kneeling position and with alternate arm and leg forwards.

Movement

Crawling forwards

The therapist positions herself in Kneeling behind the patient and grasps both his feet by the dorsum only (Figure 222).

To crawl forwards and to the right the therapist raises the patient's right leg into extension/adduction with lateral rotation. On the command '*pull*' the patient flexes, abducts and medially rotates the leg. The therapist then raises the left leg into extension/abduction with medial rotation and on the command '*pull*' the patient flexes, adducts and laterally rotates the leg.

This method is adapted to enable the patient to crawl forwards towards the left.

The patient either automatically adopts contralateral movements of the arms or is instructed to do so.

In the early stages of crawling infants keep their knees in abduction. This method of crawling may be adopted for a patient with poor balance.

Crawling backwards

The therapist positions herself as before, kneeling behind the patient, and grasps both feet ensuring that pressure is exerted on the plantar surface of the feet only.

To crawl backwards towards the right the therapist pushes the right leg into flexion/adduction with lateral rotation and on the command '*push*' the patient thrusts the leg

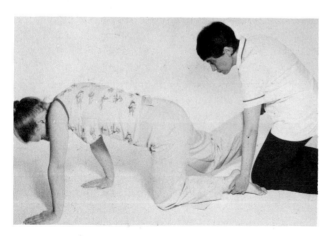

Figure 222   Resisted crawling forwards.

into extension/abduction with medial rotation. The therapist then resists the thrust of the left leg into extension/adduction with lateral rotation. This method should be adapted for crawling backwards to the left.

The patient either automatically adopts or is instructed to make contralateral movements with the arms.

These resisted movements of the legs as described can be used as resisted exercises by applying either the Repeated Contraction or Slow Reversal techniques.

KNEELING

Kneeling is a more difficult position to maintain, as the centre of gravity is raised, the base is smaller and the line of gravity falls near to the edge of the base. Developmentally the child achieves Standing and Walking before he learns to kneel and walk on his knees. However, it is usually through this position that the adult achieves Standing or raises himself from the floor into Sitting on a chair or bed. Walking on the knees is a necessary activity in some cases.

Starting position

1 The patient may be helped into Kneeling from Prone Kneeling by the therapist who takes up a position of Kneel Sitting facing the Prone Kneeling patient. The patient places his hands one at a time on the therapist's shoulders, who then raises herself into the Kneeling position moving towards the patient until they are both Kneeling facing each other, with the patient supporting himself with his hands on the therapist's shoulders and the therapist supporting the patient at waist level.
2 The patient may get himself into Kneeling by Crawling up to the wall bars and 'walking' up the bars with his hands, moving his knees towards the bars as necessary.

The patient is then taught to balance in the position by the therapist, using the head, shoulders and hips as stabilizing points.

Teaching the patient to achieve the position

Kneeling is achieved from Side Sitting, i.e. sideways with rotation, or from Kneel Sitting, a straight thrust.

From Side Sitting The patient is positioned in Kneeling either facing the wall bars which he grasps or facing a high mat, which he uses to support himself with his arms. The therapist kneels at one side and grasping the patient by the waist band (iliac crest) rotates his pelvis towards herself. The patient is then instructed to '*pull up*' and against resistance he is allowed to return to Kneeling. Gradually the therapist pulls the patient further towards the Side Sitting position and each time he returns to the starting position until he can raise himself from the floor. The patient can learn to raise himself into the Kneeling position from Side Sitting by pushing on his supporting hand and underneath leg. Obviously, if the patient is weak down one side he will find it easier if he sits towards the stronger side so that he will be supported by the stronger arm, which he can then use to push himself into Kneeling.

From Kneel Sitting The patient sits back onto his heels from Prone Kneeling and places his hands on his thighs. By thrusting with his hands, and extending his neck and hips he can raise himself into the Kneeling position. The therapist can assist by giving direction to the movement by placing one hand on the front of the patient's head and the other on one of his shoulders. She may find it necessary to help the patient to extend his hips by grasping his iliac crests or waist band.

Movement

The patient may be taught to walk on his knees against resistance, he can walk forwards or backwards, towards the right or left, or sideways in a similar manner to resisted crawling. The therapist gives resistance either at the head and shoulder or on the iliac crests.

The therapist may find it useful to give the patient shortened axillary or elbow crutches and teach balance and kneel walking on these.

From the floor to sitting on a chair/bed

Sideways with rotation

This activity is achieved through Half Kneeling. The patient takes up the Kneeling position with his stronger side against the support. The support should be large and very stable (high mat or low plinth) so that the patient will feel secure. As he gains in ability and confidence he can be taught to get into an armchair or even onto a stool, but the latter is unstable and only has a small area on which to place his buttocks. In most instances it is unsafe and unnecessary for a patient to use a stool.

From the Kneeling position the patient puts his near hand onto the high mat and taking weight through this hand he raises the ipsilateral (inside) knee and places the foot on the floor. The therapist may need to assist him to do this. The patient is taught to balance in Half Kneeling using the head, shoulder, hips, raised knee and foot as pivots for Rhythmic Stabilization.

It will be noted that in this position the

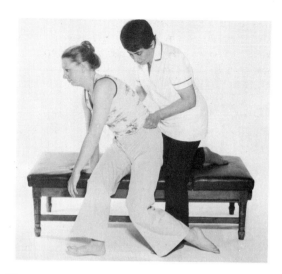

Figure 223 Assisted/resisted movement from Half Kneeling to Sitting.

patient's buttocks are level with the support. To raise himself into the Sitting position it is only necessary for him to pivot on the supporting hand, thrust with the raised leg and rotate the pelvis towards the support (Figure 223).

To assist the patient the therapist takes up a position behind him and places her nearside knee onto the high mat, ensuring that the foot that remains on the floor and the supporting knee are in the line of movement to be taken by the patient's pelvis. She then grasps the waist band of the patient's trousers. The patient and the therapist synchronize their efforts and the patient achieves the Sitting position.

This sideways movement is the basis for transfers either from Sitting through Standing or direct from Sitting to Sitting.

The reverse movement may be used to enable the patient to return to the floor. Some patients prefer to rotate the trunk through a greater range so that they can place both hands on the bed or chair arms. They then flex their knees and rotate the pelvis. At the completion of the movement the patient is kneeling facing the support rather than sideways to it.

Straight anteroposterior movement

This method may be preferred by patients who have good power in both arms.

As a preparatory exercise the patient takes up the position of Long Sitting on the mat and grasps a pair of blocks which are placed one on either side at hip level. The therapist kneels at the patient's feet and grasps them over the dorsum in such a way that she can lift them off the mat (Figure 224). The patient is instructed to raise his hips off the mat by thrusting on the blocks and the therapist raises his feet. The patient retains this position and starts to move his hips backwards and forwards. As the hips move backwards his head moves forwards, i.e. flexes, and vice versa. This rocking takes the hips through an anteroposterior arc of movement. That is, as

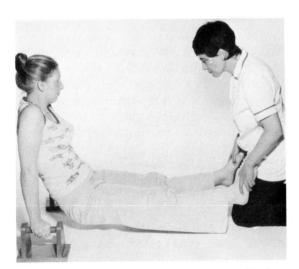

Figure 224   Assisted/resisted rocking with blocks.

the hips move backwards they are raised further from the mat, sufficient to clear a low obstacle. When resisting the forwards movement of the patient the therapist should change her grip so that she is giving pressure over the plantar surface of the feet.

To get from the floor using this method it may be necessary, certainly at first, for the movement to take place in two stages. Stage one onto a low platform or firm cushion, stage two up onto the high mat or chair. The patient sits with his back to the bed or chair, places his hands onto the support and using the same movement as previously practised, thrusts with his arms, raises his hips clear of the mat and carries them backwards onto the support (Figure 217).

Kneeling to standing

The patient takes up the Half Kneeling position,

1 Facing and supporting himself on the wall bars. The therapist stands behind the patient and places one hand on the hip of the forward leg and the other on the opposite shoulder.
2 Facing the therapist and supporting himself by placing his hands onto her shoulders. The therapist grasps the patient's waist band.

The raised knee and foot should be placed to one side, i.e. in the flexion/abduction position. (It is quite difficult for a normal individual to stand from Half Kneeling if the foot is placed directly in front of the body.)

Using the principle of maximum resistance the therapist allows the patient to stand.

Standing unaided is difficult or impossible for many patients.

Before attempting to get the patient to Stand either directly from the floor or through Sitting the therapist must ensure that he can balance in the position.

CHAPTER 27
Balance

P. J. WADDINGTON

Balance and Posture are interrelated. Depending upon the base and the position of the centre and line of gravity, a body is either balanced—in equilibrium—or not. Posture is the word used to describe any position of the human body. Some positions or postures require more muscle work to maintain than others but whatever the position, balance must be maintained otherwise the force of gravity will impose a change of posture.

The maintenance of balance is dependent on the one hand upon the integration of sensory input from exteroceptors, proprioceptors and the special senses—the eyes and the vestibular apparatus, and on the other on an integrated motor system and the basic postural reflexes. In the normal individual balance is maintained almost completely at a subconscious level. In retraining a patient's balance this fact must be considered and the patient trained to react to stimuli rather than to make a conscious, voluntary effort to maintain equilibrium. At times voluntary control will have to be exercised, but this causes the patient to be at a great disadvantage.

Balance, therefore, is the basis of all static or dynamic postures and should be considered when planning any exercise or rehabilitation programme. Its re-education should not be confined to patients with neurological conditions, as balance is frequently impaired following fractures, soft tissue lesions and surgical procedures involving the lower limb.

Balance reactions can also be used to facilitate the contraction of selected muscle groups and as part of a muscle strengthening programme.

There are two approaches to balance both of which are necessary for normal function—*static balance* and *dynamic balance*.

Static balance

This approach is based upon P.N.F. principles and techniques.

Static balance is the rigid stability of one part of the body on another and is based upon isometric and co-contraction of muscle. The Rhythmic Stabilization technique and the irradiation principle are used to develop a contraction of postural muscles. These techniques may be used in any position. They are frequently combined with compression to stimulate postural reflexes.

As a general principle balance is developed progressively by moving from the most stable to the least stable position, for example from Forearm Support Prone Lying to Standing with sticks.

Stability and control of the head should be established first as it is vital in all positions. Strong neck muscles can then be used to reinforce muscle contraction elsewhere. Assessment of the patient's muscle strength will

236

guide the therapist in the application of the irradiation principle. NOTE: the possibilities of associated reactions and an undesirable increase in tone must always be considered. However, this method is useful with patients who are hypotonic or ataxic.

Application

As indicated above, positions for the retraining of balance are selected on the basis of progression from the easy to the more difficult.

Positions Forearm Support Prone Lying
Forearm Support Prone Kneeling
Prone Kneeling
Reach Grasp Kneeling
Half Kneeling
Sitting
Walk Standing
Standing

Although in the normal development of the child, standing is achieved before kneeling, for the adult, Kneeling, and certainly Reach Grasp Kneeling are frequently easier to maintain than Standing. If required as a progression shortened crutches may be used for support in kneeling.

In Standing and Walk Standing the patient may be progressed from using parallel bars, through the range of walking aids to Standing unaided.

Resistance is applied to all the components needed to maintain a particular position. Selection is made from the following:

Head
Shoulders
Pelvis
Knees
Toes for gripping the floor
Hands for gripping a support or a walking
   aid

A slow increase of alternating resistance is used to build up a co-contraction, i.e. Rhythmic Stabilization. The direction of the resistance will vary with the point selected, for example:

1   The pelvis
    a   Forwards and backwards
    b   Laterally
    c   Diagonally
    d   Rotation
2   The knee
    Forwards and backwards

A combination of stabilizing points may be used to advantage, e.g. the shoulder and the pelvis, the head and the pelvis, the pelvis and the knee.

In some situations the principles of maximal resistance are used to stimulate a unilateral isometric contraction instead of a co-contraction; this is of particular value when working to obtain extension of the cervical spine in Forearm Support Prone Lying.

Dynamic balance

This approach is based upon Bobath principles and techniques.

The body, unless it is fully supported and relaxed, is in a constant state of adjustment to maintain its posture and its equilibrium. The forces tending to upset this balance may vary in strength from the infinitesimal to sufficient to completely upset the individual's equilibrium so that he falls to the ground. Consequently, the body's reactions to maintain its equilibrium will vary in degree. For example, the amount of adjustment will be greater and more obvious when an individual slips on an ice-covered road than when he raises his hand to his mouth. The normal individual will find the former a difficult if not impossible exercise in regaining balance but he will not even be aware of the adjustments he makes when eating. However, raising the hand to the mouth will prove a severe test of balance for a paraplegic patient early in his rehabilitation, while he is still learning to compensate for the loss of sensory input from below the lesion.

At the level of minor adjustments, the muscles may be working either isometrically or isotonically but when larger adjustments are necessary the type of muscle work will become definitely isotonic. If one had to try to clarify this it is easier to work with the concept of static balance as being isometric and dynamic balance as being isotonic contraction.

It is convenient to think of these balance reactions as occurring in two ways:

a An adjustment in tone to maintain a position.
b An adjustment in posture to maintain or regain balance. This can involve either movements designed to keep the individual in more or less the same place, or those in which the base is moved.

Maintenance of position

This method, unlike Rhythmic Stabilization, allows for a little movement.

The patient is instructed to maintain the position, for example, Prone Kneeling, Kneeling, Sitting or Standing against the therapist's tapping technique. This technique simply consists of tapping the patient's shoulders or thorax at shoulder level, first in one direction and then in the other. The tap should be strong enough to cause the patient to adjust his muscle tone but not strong enough to make him change his position. For example, when he is Standing, a tap on the patient's back causing the body to move slightly forwards

will cause the calf muscles to contract, a tap in the opposite direction will cause a contraction of the anterior tibial muscles. This is obviously an oversimplification as changes in muscle tone will occur elsewhere, particularly in the feet.

Maintaining or regaining balance

It has been said that our whole life consists of constantly regaining our balance. We are never static. One view of walking is that it is simply a transferring of weight forwards and that the leg moves to regain balance.

Balance reactions are immediate and reliable and are not learned at a voluntary level. Therefore, the therapist does not instruct the patient in how to react but puts him into such a situation that he has to react to maintain or regain his balance. It is usually a wise precaution to explain to the patient that you are going to work on balance otherwise he may get very frustrated as most patients expect to be told what to do in the form of a definite task or exercise. Further instruction would destroy the patient's ability to react spontaneously.

The therapist must know the normal balance reactions, so that she will be able to recognize the abnormal and also so that she can facilitate normal reactions where they are absent.

An interesting point to note is the change of tone in a limb before it actually moves. The student can easily try this for herself. In the Prone Kneeling position do not move but think about lifting one hand from the ground and note the change of pressure and of tone. Without this preparation movement would not be possible.

The use of a moving support is valuable in some positions to facilitate movement and in others can be related to balance maintenance in such common situations as riding in a bus or car or on a bicycle or ship.

There are three basic types of movable support, *a balance board* which can vary in size from the usual wobble board (Chapter 3) to a polished piece of wood 2000 mm long and 610 mm wide with a rocker at either end: *a roll* which can be made of a cardboard tube, as used in carpets, is padded and covered with plastic and *large inflated balls* of varying size and type.

Lying   This position is not usually associated with problems of balance but if the therapist wishes to stimulate movement, particularly trunk movement, the patient can be placed in Lying on a polished balance board. The therapist controls the board from one end and tilts it so that the patient has to react to remain on the board. From the age of 6 months a child will try to stay on the board. The disadvantage is that it is difficult for the therapist to control both the board and the patient.

Rolling a patient on a mat may be used as a method for reducing tone. A pathological pattern and the accompanying hypertonus is a complete entity. General reduction in tone as a preparation for movement starts with efforts to produce symmetry and trunk rotation. Trunk rotation is lost in patients with Parkinson's disease and trunk rolling can be used followed by the Rhythm technique (Chapter 25). Following the reduction in tone, active balance reactions occur. These movements, in themselves, tend to reduce tone still further. Even where hypertonus is not a problem, balance reactions in Lying may be used as a form of exercise. There are several ways of producing trunk rotation passively but to activate the patient the following methods will form a basis for stimulating activity.

The patient is placed in Lying with the therapist Kneel Sitting so that the patient's head is resting on her knees. The patient's arms, when possible, are placed in the flexion/abduction/lateral rotation position which is a reflex inhibitory pattern, i.e. a position opposite to the basic pathological pattern of spasticity. This position in itself will tend to reduce tone as a preparation for movement. The therapist places her hands high on the patient's scapulae and rolls him first to one side and then to the other. Once the patient begins to show some movement more time is spent with him in the Side Lying position. The therapist slightly adjusts the patient's position, constantly putting him off balance so that he has to move either his trunk or the upper leg to regain his equilibrium (Figure 225).

This method can prove impossible if the patient is too heavy to move from the Supine

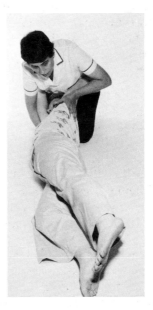

Figure 225   Balance reactions in Side Lying.

position. When this is so, Side Lying can be used as a starting position to activate balance reactions. Also Side Lying is useful as the labyrinthine reflexes are not stimulated in that position and if care is taken to ensure that the head and neck are aligned neither are the asymmetrical tonic neck reflexes.

Prone Kneeling (normal reactions)   The patient takes up the Prone Kneeling position. The therapist raises one of his limbs to elicit balance reactions. When the arm is used it should be kept laterally rotated and the thumb extended. There are three basic types of reaction.

a   When a normal limb is raised and moved

slowly, without the help of the patient, it will feel light and easy to move and the body will adapt itself easily to maintain its balance.

The next two types of reaction occur when enough force is applied to endanger the patient's equilibrium. Each person, depending upon his physical strength and possibly his personality, will have an automatic preference for one or the other.

b   The patient tries to maintain his position by developing a co-contraction, i.e. static balance. This is usually adequate up to a certain point, at which the patient can no longer resist and he collapses onto the mat.

c   The patient moves another limb to maintain his equilibrium. If the therapist moves one limb into abduction the patient will raise his contralateral limb (Figure 226). If she adducts the limb the patient will raise the ipsilateral limb (Figure 227).

Some people will crawl about following the

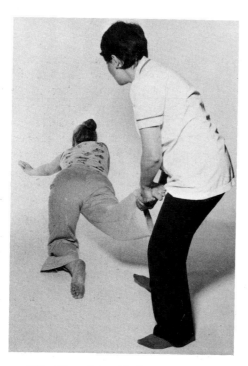

Figure 226   Contralateral balance reaction in Prone Kneeling.

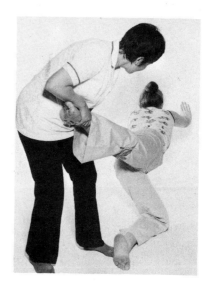

Figure 227   Ipsilateral balance reaction in Prone Kneeling.

limb that is being moved. This really does not come under the narrow heading of balance reactions. Patients who do this are obviously quite safe in Prone Kneeling. If the therapist wishes to use these equilibrium reactions as a form of exercise for such patients she may have to give him a further explanation of what is required.

Kneeling (normal reactions)
a   Weight transference forwards—the therapist Kneels in front of the patient and displaces his weight forwards holding him at waist level. The patient reacts by abducting the arms and extending the fingers and thumb, flexing the knees and plantarflexing at the ankle (Figure 228).
b   Weight transference laterally—again the arms abduct and the fingers extend. The non-weight bearing leg is abducted (Figure 229).

Standing (normal reactions)   The therapist,

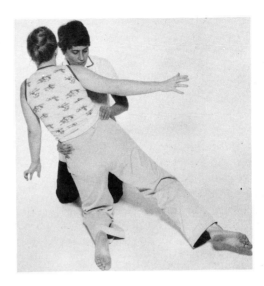

Figure 229 Balance reaction in Kneeling—weight transferred laterally.

standing behind the patient, can hold the patient at the pelvis (thumbs inserted into waist band or belt), shoulders, knees or head. Obviously the patient feels safer if held at the pelvis and in practice this is usually done as the majority of patients are apprehensive. Again a judgement has to be made as the patient must not feel too secure.

These balance reactions may be done with either the patient standing on a mat or on the floor. Many nervous patients prefer to stand on the mat although a thick mat forms a less secure base and may be selected by the therapist for that reason, i.e. to elicit a reaction.

The therapist may decide to cause a patient either to take weight on an affected leg or to move it.

a   Weight transference backwards—causes dorsiflexion at the ankle. Further disturbance will cause the patient to take a step backwards

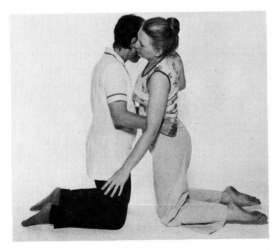

Figure 228 Balance reaction in Kneeling—weight transferred forwards.

if he is prevented from doing this by the therapist placing a foot at the back of his heels, the patient will bend forward from the waist and hips raising the arms forwards simultaneously. Some people may prefer this reaction in any situation.

b Weight transference forwards—will cause the patient to stand on his toes. If this is the reaction required the therapist would be better standing facing the patient. Further transference of weight forwards will cause the patient to step.

c Weight transference laterally—the therapist transfers the patient's weight onto one foot, the patient either abducts the non-weight bearing leg or crosses it in front of the weight

bearing leg (Figure 230). The first reaction may be followed by the second. If the weight is then transferred in the opposite direction the leg will return to the starting position. This alternating weight transfer may be done rhythmically causing the moving leg to react repeatedly.

Standing on one foot (normal reactions) The therapist asks the patient to stand on one foot. She grasps the raised leg taking the foot in one hand, using the other to grasp the posterior aspect of the leg just below the knee. It is usually preferable to keep the patient's knee flexed.
Reactions:

a Slight movement of the raised leg by the therapist will result in considerable activity of the standing foot which will remain stationary (Figure 231).

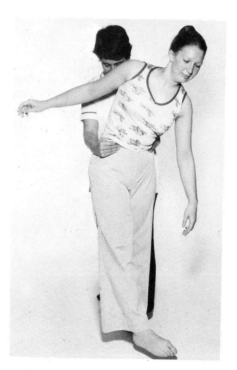

Figure 230 Balance reaction in Standing—weight transferred laterally.

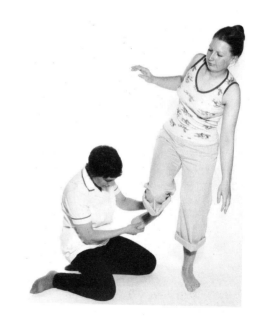

Figure 231 Balance reaction—Standing on one foot.

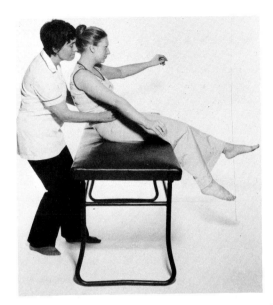

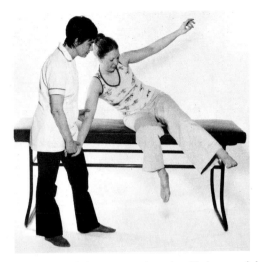

Figure 233 Balance reaction in Sitting—weight transferred laterally.

Figure 232 Balance reaction in Sitting—weight transferred backwards.

b Further movement of the raised leg by the therapist will cause the patient to move, either by doing a heel–toe pivot or by hopping. Again the normal person will have his own preferred reaction.

Sitting The patient sits so that the feet are unsupported.

a Weight transference backwards—the therapist may stand either behind or in front of the patient grasping the pelvis. The patient reacts by extending the knees (Figure 232).
b Weight transference forwards—the therapist stands facing the patient and grasps the pelvis. The patient reacts by further flexion of the knees.
c Weight transference laterally—the patient's weight may be transferred by moving either the arm or the leg. The weight is transferred laterally initially (Figure 233). Once

the patient's balance reactions are facilitated many movements can be elicited by further movements of the limb. These movements involve a considerable amount of effort on the patient's part to maintain his balance. Some individuals react by resisting the therapist and so develop a co-contraction.

NOTE: A knowledge of normal balance reactions enables the therapist to use these not only in the retraining of balance and thus confidence in the patient but also as a means of eliciting a contraction in exercising specific muscle groups.

Protective extension reaction of the arms

If balance reactions fail, protective extension (saving reactions) of the arms is one of the most important reactions. In patients with central nervous system damage it may be necessary to facilitate this reaction either in infants and children who have never developed it or in adults where it has been disturbed. Again these techniques may be used as a means of eliciting a muscle contraction.

Such discussion moves into the area of normal development and the treatment of specific conditions which are outside the scope of this book.

It may be useful to indicate some of the ways in which this reaction may be elicited.

1   The patient is placed in the Sitting position.

a   The therapist holds the unaffected arm and transfers the patient's weight sideways towards the affected side.

b   The therapist holds the affected arm by *either* using one of her hands to keep the patient's wrist and fingers extended and her thumb abducted and the other hand to control the elbow, *or* using both hands to maintain the extended wrist and fingers and the abducted thumb. Some of the patient's weight is then transferred through the affected arm. The therapist may then use a pull–push technique in the long axis of the limb to facilitate the protective extension reaction.

2   The patient is placed in the Prone Kneeling position. The therapist raises either one or *both* of the patient's arms by grasping at the shoulder and releases her grasp.

3   The patient is Standing. The therapist stands facing the patient and grasps the hands, palm-to-palm, keeping the wrists extended and when possible the thumbs abducted. The patient's arms are raised into the Reach position and the therapist gently pulls the patient towards herself so transferring his weight forwards. The push–pull technique through the longitudinal axis of the arm may again be used to elicit a response.

The reactions of some patients who have made an almost complete recovery may be speeded up by pushing them forwards onto a plinth or wall. The therapist may keep control of the patient by retaining her hold of one arm.

CHAPTER 28
Gait

P. J. WADDINGTON

The problems presented by the patient who is unable to walk, but has the potential to do so, and by the patient with abnormal gait are manifold. The assessment of each patient must be the basis for satisfactory treatment. The therapist who looks at the problem from more than one standpoint will have a better chance of solving it.

Walking is a complex combination of balance and coordinated muscle contraction based on normal tone and power and on sensory input. Too much time can be spent in instructing the patient to perform specific movements at a conscious voluntary level. Walking is a reflex activity which takes place at a subconscious level. It is obvious that the patient who is being instructed in the use of a walking aid will have to know what is expected of him but the aim is to produce a conditioned reflex so that the aid becomes part of his normal walking pattern.

When possible, walking should be trained as a reaction to sensory input based on normal muscle tone and the use of specific instructions about localized movement should be reduced to a minimum. With some patients the difficulty facing the therapist is to decide at what point the efforts at attempting to train a normal gait pattern should be abandoned and the patient and the therapist should accept an abnormal pattern and/or the introduction of an appliance or a walking aid,

i.e. to consider walking merely as a means by which the patient can have some degree of independence in moving from place to place.

Standing balance is an essential prerequisite to walking. Time spent in gaining this before walking is attempted is vital as the patient who is unsure of his balance will be tense and afraid to move.

Walking aids feature in most gait training programmes (Chapter 11) as:

a A progression from parallel bars to the minimum necessary to enable patients who have been immobile for a period to develop their full potential.

b A temporary measure, for example, for patients with lower limb injuries who have to be non-weight bearing or partial weight bearing for a limited period.

c A permanent aid for patients with no possibility of improvement.

The usual type of stick or crutch has been found to have an undesirable effect on some patients with Cerebral Palsy. The position in which sticks are usually held emphasizes the spastic pattern. In such cases the use of poles about half as long again as normal sticks may be used to help the patient's balance. To grip the poles, which he is encouraged to keep well out to the side, the patient's arms will be laterally rotated and the forearms supinated (Figure 234). The therapist can control the

245

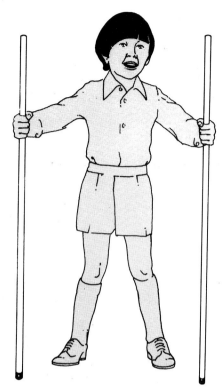

Figure 234   Standing—using poles to aid balance.

poles from the top when standing behind the patient.

Gait training is not complete until the patient can walk forwards, backwards, sideways and in a diagonal direction. To be fully independent the patient also needs to be able to negotiate stairs, slopes, uneven surfaces and other people moving or standing in close proximity.

Resisted walking

The therapist selects the walking aid which will enable the patient to concentrate his maximum effort on walking. The parallel bars are frequently used in the early stages of training.

Resisted walking may be selected with one of two aims.

1   As a means whereby the therapist can give as much sensory information as possible while allowing the patient to move smoothly through the walking pattern which in itself establishes his sensory image of walking.

2   As a means of increasing joint range, particularly at the knee and ankle, when it is limited following injury. The therapist encourages the patient, usually within the parallel bars, to work against a high degree of resistance thus exaggerating the walking pattern and the power of contraction of the muscles bringing about the movement.

Method

A   The therapist ensures that the patient has adequate balance.

B   She also ensures that he is in control of the walking aid and using it effectively. The patient's grip is tested and reinforced. The therapist grasps the patient's fingers with one hand and his thumb with the other. She then exerts resistance to the grip until the patient is working maximally. The grip must not be broken. Frequently when patients first use a crutch or stick they fail to exert enough downward pressure. In some instances they simply lift the aid off the floor. This downward pressure and stability can be facilitated, by the therapist tapping the stick about halfway down, first from one side and then from the other in quick succession. Alternatively she may place her hand over the patient's and try to lift the aid off the floor. The command will be '*Don't let me move it*'.

C   The therapist stands in front of the patient if he is to walk forwards (Figure 235) or

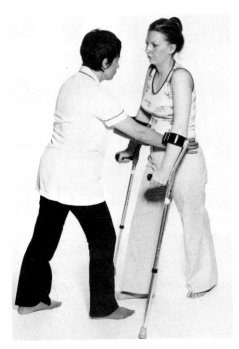

Figure 235 Resisted walking.

ward pressure is again given and the cycle repeated.

When resisted walking is being used to increase range of movement at a particular joint emphasis is placed on resisting the forward movement. The patient may appear to be moving in slow motion and feel that he is walking uphill.

Facilitating normal gait through trunk rotation

Trunk rotation is the foundation of correct walking and when this is absent an abnormal pattern results. Trunk rotation is lost in patients with rigidity, e.g. with Parkinsonism and in patients who hold themselves stiff usually through fear and lack of confidence in their ability to walk following injury. It is not unusual when young children are learning to march to see one, who perhaps is a little uncoordinated, making a great effort, the result being ipsilateral instead of contralateral movements of both the arms and the legs.

Method

Trunk rotation can be imposed upon the patient when he is walking by the therapist who either rotates the trunk directly by using the pelvis or shoulder girdle, or indirectly through the arms. It is usual only to use these techniques when the patient is walking forwards.

Both these methods when first used by the therapist may pose a rather difficult problem of coordination.

Directly The therapist stands behind the patient. In the early stages of using this technique it is advisable to establish with the patient which leg he is going to move forwards initially, because the therapist needs to

behind him if he is to walk backwards. She places her hands on his iliac crests with either forward or backward pressure as necessary to give exteroceptive stimulation for the direction of movement and in preparation for resisting walking. The therapist may find it useful to slip her thumbs into the waist band of the patient's trousers, through which, if necessary, she can control the pelvis.

D As the patient walks the therapist exerts firm pressure downwards at every step on 'heel strike' to facilitate the postural reflexes.

E She then ensures that the patient transfers his weight into the now standing leg simultaneously resisting or assisting the progression of the moving leg.

F On 'heel strike' of the other leg, down-be in position before the patient starts to walk as she has to change her manual contacts quickly. The patient takes the first step with his right leg.

1 The pelvis: The therapist places her right hand over the anterior superior iliac spine and her left on the posterior aspect of the iliac crest. As the patient moves his right leg forwards she pulls backwards with her right hand and pushes forwards with her left hand. This has the effect of rotating the trunk to the right and the left arm swings forwards. She reverses the position of her hands and the pulling and pushing movements with each step.

2 The shoulders: The therapist places her right hand on the front of the patient's right shoulder and her left hand on the back of the patient's left shoulder. As the patient moves his right leg forwards she pulls backwards with her right hand and pushes forwards with her left hand. As with the pelvic control this has the effect of rotating the patient's trunk to the right and the left arm swings forwards. She reverses the position of her hands and the

pulling and pushing movements with each step.

The therapist's selection of either the pelvis or shoulders as a point of control will depend upon the patient's response and the relative height of the patient and the therapist.

Indirectly The therapist obtains a pair of wooden sticks or poles of similar length and stands in front of the patient facing him. She holds one end of each stick and the patient holds the other end. They both allow their arms to hang loosely at their sides. Having established with the patient the leg with which he will take his first step, e.g. the right, she prepares to step backwards simultaneously with her left leg. The therapist instructs the patient to start walking; she walks backwards keeping in step and at the same time moving the patient's arms contralaterally through the sticks. Vigorous, large-range movement of the arms imposes trunk rotation. If necessary the therapist, through the sticks, can help the patient to keep his balance.

Bibliography

ADAMS, R.C., DANIEL, A.N. & PULLMAN, L. (1972) *Games, Sports & Exercises for the Physically Handicapped*, Lea & Febiger: Philadelphia

AMERICAN ACADEMY OF ORTHOPAEDIC SURGEONS (1965) *Joint Motion*, reprinted (by Permission) by The British Orthopaedic Association 1966.

CARLSÖÖ, S. (1972) *How Man Moves* translated by William P. Michael, Heinemann: London

CASH, J.E. (1974) Editor *Neurology for Physiotherapists*, Chapters 1–6 by Helen W. Atkinson, Faber & Faber: London

CHARTERED SOCIETY OF PHYSIOTHERAPY (1975) *Handling the Handicapped*, Woodhead-Faulkner: Cambridge

COLSON, J. (1969) *Progressive Exercise Therapy*, John Wright & Sons: Bristol

FREEMAN, I. (1967) *Physics made Simple*, W.H. Allen: London

FREEMAN, M.A.R. (1965) Co-ordination exercises in the treatment of functional instability of the foot, *Physiotherapy*, **51**, 12

GANONG, W.F. (1969) *Review of Medical Physiology*, Lange Medical Publications: Los Detos, California

GARDNER, D. (1971) *The Principles of Exercise Therapy*, G. Bell & Sons: London

GASKELL, D.V. & WEBBER, B.A. (1980) *The Brompton Hospital Guide to Physiotherapy*, 4th ed., Blackwell Scientific Publications: Oxford

HOLLIS, M. & ROPER, M.H.S. (1965) *Suspension Therapy*, Baillière Tindall & Cassell: London

ILLINGWORTH, R.S. (1973) *Basic Developmental Screening*, Blackwell Scientific Publications: Oxford

KABAT, H. (1958) Proprioception in therapeutic exercise in *Therapeutic Exercise*, Editor S. Licht, Elizabeth Licht, New Haven, Connecticut

KNOTT, M. & VOSS, D. (1968) *Proprioceptive Neuromuscular Facilitation—Patterns and Techniques*, 2nd ed., Hoeber Medical Division, Harper & Row: London

MACDONALD, F.A. (1974) *Mechanics for Movement*, G. Bell & Sons: London

McLEOD, J., FRENCH, E.B. & MUNRO, J.F. (1974) *Introduction to Clinical Examination*, Churchill Livingstone: Edinburgh

MEDICAL RESEARCH COUNCIL (1972) *Aids to the Investigation of Peripheral Nerve Injuries*, HMSO: London

MENNELL, J.B. (1967) *Physical Treatment by Movement Manipulation and Massage*, J. & A. Churchill: Edinburgh

MITCHELL, L. (1900) *Physiological Relaxation*

MORGAN, R.E. & ADAMSON, G.T. (1961) *Circuit Training*, G. Bell & Sons: London

NEUMANN-NEURODE (1967) *Baby Gymnastics*, Revised by W. Kaiser, Pergamon Press: Oxford

WELLS, K.F. (1966) *Kinesiology*, W.B. Saunders Co: Philadelphia

WILLIAMS, M. & LISSNER, H.R. (1969) *Biomechanics of Human Motion*, W.B. Saunders Co: Philadelphia

Index